Exercise Prescription Case Studies for Healthy Populations

Exercise Prescription Case Studies for Healthy Populations

Revised First Edition

Bradley R.A Wilson, Ph.D. and Matthew D. McCabe, Ph.D.

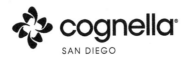

SAN DIEGO

Bassim Hamadeh, CEO and Publisher
Carrie Baarns, Manager, Revisions and Author Care
Kaela Martin, Project Editor
Abbey Hastings, Production Editor
Emely Villavicencio, Senior Graphic Designer
Alexa Lucido, Licensing Manager
Natalie Piccotti, Director of Marketing
Kassie Graves, Senior Vice President, Editorial
Jamie Giganti, Director of Academic Publishing

Cover images: Copyright © 2016 Depositphotos/Rawpixel.
    Copyright © 2017 Depositphotos/Rawpixel.
    Copyright © 2017 Depositphotos/Rawpixel.
    Copyright © 2017 Depositphotos/Rawpixel.
    Copyright © 2017 Depositphotos/Rawpixel.
    Copyright © 2017 iStockphoto LP/gradyreese.

Printed in the United States of America.

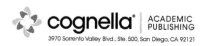
cognella® | ACADEMIC PUBLISHING
3970 Sorrento Valley Blvd., Ste. 500, San Diego, CA 92121

To my children Alexa, Nicholas, and Olivia for being the light of my life.
—BW

To Forrest, Anita, Mark, and Andrea McCabe for their continuous love and support.
—MM

Brief Contents

Detailed Contents

Preface

We wrote this book to provide students with the opportunity to apply the knowledge they have learned in classes to situations they are likely to encounter when writing exercise prescriptions in actual settings. Because writing exercise prescriptions uses scientific information learned in many different courses in an exercise curriculum, the purpose of this book is not to teach students all of the concepts involved with writing exercise prescriptions, but rather to review and synthesize the information learned into practical applications. Additionally, completing the case studies in this book will help prepare students for the ACSM Certified Exercise Physiologist® exam.

The case studies presented closely follow the guidelines established by the American College of Sports Medicine. These are clearly outlined in *ACSM's Guidelines for Exercise Testing and Prescription*, 11th edition. Because this book states very specific information about conducting exercise tests, interpreting the results, and writing exercise prescriptions, we believe that all exercise students and exercise physiologists should have the most recent edition as part of their library and regularly use it as a reference. Although the guidelines book is very detailed and concise, it does not provide all of the background explanations required for good student understanding. Therefore, other resources are required to provide that information. Our book is an effort to fill in some of those gaps.

The focus of this book is on apparently healthy individuals and includes children, adolescents, older adults, and pregnant women. To begin learning about how to write an exercise prescription it is logical to start with individuals who have no known chronic diseases. Once a good understanding of the process for healthy individuals is obtained, the next steps would then be writing prescriptions for those with controlled diseases, followed by clinical populations.

This book presents case studies that involve the continuum of information from screenings to writing the exercise prescriptions. Although the focus is on healthy individuals, it is a reality that some people who appear healthy may not actually be healthy. Therefore, Chapter 4 includes some concepts of clinical exercise testing. This information will help students understand the individuals who may come to them for an exercise prescription after completing a clinical exercise test that found them to be healthy, or in other words, negative for cardiovascular disease.

Further, the earlier book chapters each focus on one different component of the exercise prescription process until the last chapter, which pulls together all of the components into comprehensive case studies. This will help students break the process into pieces and then put them all together. We hope that students will find the case studies interesting and enjoyable. In the end students should have better skills for developing exercise programs to score well on certification exams and meet the specific needs of their clients.

Acknowledgments

The authors would like to offer their gratitude to all of the exercise professionals who have contributed to the knowledge for writing exercise prescriptions over the years. Without them, there would be no reason to write this book. Special credit goes to the past and current leaders of the American College of Sports Medicine for establishing and updating the guidelines used for safe exercise testing and prescription.

We would also like to recognize Cognella Academic Publishers for helping us to make this book a reality. Our sincere appreciation is extended to Jennifer Codner, Michelle Piehl, and Jeanine Rees for their exceptional guidance and continual support.

Screening for Exercise Participation

INTRODUCTION

WHILE MOST PEOPLE are aware that exercise is beneficial for health, not exercising properly can result in injuries and health complications. Therefore, it is prudent to evaluate a person's health before completing an exercise test or prescribing an exercise program. This chapter includes four case studies that provide students with an opportunity to think through the steps necessary to determine whether a person is healthy enough to exercise safely. Some may need to get medical clearance while others may be able to exercise right away. Determining whether a client or patient needs medical clearance before beginning an exercise program is a very important responsibility for exercise professionals. Following the appropriate guidelines is crucial for good practice and promoting safe and effective exercise.

Completing any case study requires a certain level of knowledge. Before starting the case studies in this chapter, students must know about cardiovascular, metabolic, and renal diseases including their major signs and symptoms.[1] This information is critical to determining whether medical clearance is recommended before beginning or continuing exercise programs at moderate and vigorous intensities.

Two different screening procedures are reviewed using a case study approach. One is the updated Physical Activity Readiness Questionnaire (PAR-Q+), which was developed as a self-screening instrument.[2] The PAR-Q+ is evidence based and is intended to be comprehendible for the general population and reduce the barriers to exercise participation. The second screening is the American College of Sports Medicine's (ACSM) Preparticipation Screening Algorithm.[3] The second method requires more technical knowledge and is widely used by exercise professionals, especially in health-related fitness facilities.

The purpose of this chapter is to teach students how to apply their knowledge of disease and exercise to determine who can exercise safely. On completion of the case studies students will be able to:

1. Assist a client on how to complete the PAR-Q+
2. Interpret the results of the PAR-Q+
3. Assist a client on how to complete the ePARmed-X+

4. Explain the results of the ePARmed-X+
5. Determine if a client should consult a physician before beginning a physical activity program based on the results of the PAR-Q+
6. Evaluate a client's symptoms for cardiovascular, metabolic, and renal diseases
7. Analyze a client's current physical activity status
8. Assess a client's known medical conditions
9. Determine whether a client should consult a physician before beginning a moderate or vigorous physical activity program based on the results of the ACSM Screening Algorithm

SELF-GUIDED SCREENING

The PAR-Q+ is a prescreening instrument that can be used by the general population to determine if an individual is healthy enough to exercise safely.[4] The initial questions, seven in number, are written to be comprehensible by non–exercise professionals. The questions do not use technical or scientific terms that most people would not understand. People who answer "no" to all seven questions can feel comfortable that it is safe for them to become more physically active. However, if at least one question is answered as "yes," then pages 2 and 3 must be completed.

Many non–exercise professionals may not understand all of the terminology used in the follow-up questions. If a person has a specific condition and has discussed it with a physician, then it would be clear when "yes" should be checked. On the other hand, if a person has never had a condition and had not discussed it with a physician, the likelihood of that person understanding the question would be less. Therefore, some people may need assistance from an exercise professional when completing pages 2 and 3.

People who answer "no" to all questions on pages 2 and 3 are ready to become more physically active. Those who answer "yes" to one or more follow-up questions must complete the ePARmed-X+ on the website www.eparmedx.com.[5] Most non–exercise professionals will need to consult a qualified exercise professional for assistance in answering these questions because they are more technical in nature.

It should be noted that on completion of the PAR-Q+ the recommendation will be either to consult a physician before becoming more physically active or that it is safe to become more physically active. The level of physical activity that is safe and recommended will depend on the person's previous activity level. Sedentary people should begin with low to moderate intensity exercise. Those who have been exercising at moderate levels can progress to vigorous exercise. Exercisers who are older than 45 years of age and have been exercising at moderate levels should consult a qualified exercise professional before beginning a vigorous exercise program.

PROFESSIONALLY GUIDED SCREENING

Certified exercise physiologists should screen their clients by using the ACSM Preparticipation Screening Algorithm, which is based on current exercise participation; known cardiovascular, metabolic, and renal disease; and signs or symptoms of cardiovascular, metabolic, and renal disease.[6] In short, if an exercise physiologist finds that a client has a known cardiovascular, metabolic, or renal disease, is a regular, moderate exerciser, and is asymptomatic medical clearance is needed only when the client wants to complete exercise of vigorous intensity and has not been medically cleared within the last 12 months.

To use this algorithm exercise physiologists must know the signs and symptoms of cardiovascular, metabolic, and renal disease. One of the most common symptoms is anginal (ischemic) chest pain, which must be distinguished from nonanginal chest pain. Typical anginal chest pain is brought on by stress, including exercise. Angina manifests as a pressure, burning pain sensation as opposed to a sharp stabbing pain. Although often called chest pain, it can radiate into the arms, shoulders, neck, and jaw. Further, exercise physiologists should be aware of how angina typically manifests in men and women. In men, angina often presents as crushing substernal chest pain that radiates to the neck, jaw, upper back, and arms. In women, angina may present as feelings of nausea and fatigue. This type of pain is indicative of reduced blood flow to the heart muscle.

Other signs and symptoms of cardiovascular, metabolic, and renal disease that are caused by the inability of the heart to pump and distribute sufficient oxygenated blood include the following. Dizziness and loss of consciousness (syncope) during exercise is an indication of insufficient blood flow to the brain. Pain in the legs during mild exertion and made worse with greater exertion is called claudication. The pain is generally caused by insufficient blood flow to the working muscles.

Some signs and symptoms affect breathing and are often due to left ventricular dysfunction. Shortness of breath or dyspnea is expected with strenuous exercise but not during mild exercise or rest. Unusual shortness of breath of this type is found in respiratory and left ventricular diseases. Shortness of breath at rest while lying down is orthopnea. When shortness of breath occurs at night while sleeping, it is called paroxysmal nocturnal dyspnea. Shortness of breath and unusual fatigue during typical activities of daily living can also indicate cardiovascular or metabolic disease.

Cardiovascular, metabolic, and renal disease signs and symptoms also include ankle edema, heart palpitations, and heart murmur. Ankle edema occurs when the body is unable to pump fluid back to the heart sufficiently. It is important to note that ankle edema may be due to a previous orthopedic injury. Therefore, exercise professionals should examine for bilateral "pitting" ankle edema. Further, unilateral ankle edema may due to venous insufficiency, which is a sign of cardiovascular disease. Heart palpitations are irregular heart rhythms that are usually noticed as a thump in the heart or fast heart rates. Heart murmurs are usually due to valve disorders.

The important reasons for knowing the signs and symptoms of cardiovascular, metabolic, and renal disease are to make note of them and determine if they are due to disease or other causes. Given that exercise physiologists do not make medical diagnoses or medical judgments, whenever the exercise physiologist doubts the origin of signs and symptoms, it is always best to err on the side of caution and recommend medical clearance. Medical referrals are needed to determine the cause, and exercise participation should be delayed until the cause is found. The first step in the ACSM preparticipation screening algorithm is to assess these signs and symptoms. If one or more are present the client must seek medical clearance before being tested or beginning an exercise program.

If no signs and symptoms of cardiovascular, metabolic, and renal disease are found the second step is to determine the client's current exercise status. To be considered as one who participates in regular exercise the client must be currently participating in a planned and structured program of at least moderate intensity for at least 30 minutes per day, at least three times per week for at least the last three months.

The third step is to consider known disease or medical conditions. If the client has been participating in a regular exercise program and has a known medical condition the exercise program can be continued at low to moderate intensities. If the client wants to progress to vigorous activities, medical clearance is recommended before increasing the intensity of work. If the client has not been participating in a regular exercise program, then medical screening is recommended before beginning any exercise program.

SUMMARY

As a first step all exercise professionals must know how to determine who can exercise safely. The PAR-Q+ and the ACSM preparticipation screening algorithm are two methods for making this determination. The following case studies will help students apply their knowledge and determine whether the client needs medical screening before beginning an exercise program.

Demonstration Case Study 1.1

PAR-Q+

Julie is a 53-year-old woman who has decided to begin an exercise program. She has participated in minimal physical activity throughout her life and has heard so much about the benefits of exercise that she started to talk with others about getting started. Keisha, a friend who exercises regularly, told her that she should make sure she is healthy enough to exercise and she should use an instrument called the PAR-Q+ because she can do it on her own. After searching online Julie found the site for the PAR-Q+ at http://eparmedx.com. Then she clicked on "Take the PAR-Q+ Survey NOW." The first question popped up and she noticed there were estimated to be eight questions. She answered "no" to the first two questions. The third question asked about dizziness, and because she has unexplained dizziness when standing up too quickly she answered "yes." The next screen said her survey was complete and she should now take the ePARmed-X+ survey.

So she clicked on the "Complete" button and was presented with a new page of directions. She then clicked on "Take the ePARmed-X+ Survey Now" and the first of an estimated 11 questions appeared. After answering "no" to the first two questions she was presented with a long list of medical conditions, most of which she did not really understand. So she clicked on "Other Diagnosed Medical Condition Not Listed OR UNKNOWN." The next page directed her to see a qualified exercise professional or her physician. She was trying to avoid making a doctor's appointment so she called her friend Keisha. Keisha said she has a personal trainer named Maria and it might be good to talk with her. Julie then made an appointment with Maria.

When Julie and Maria met, Maria pulled out a paper copy of the PAR-Q+. It was four pages long. The first page had seven questions and it looked like what she completed online, at least the first three questions that she actually saw. She again answered "yes" to the third question about dizziness and "no" to the rest. Maria said that because she answered "yes" to one question she needed to complete the 10 questions on the next two pages. Julie noticed that if she did not answer "no" to one of those 10 questions she would have to answer two to five additional questions. However, she did honestly answer "no" to all 10 and proceeded to page 4, where it indicated that she was ready to become more physically active and therefore she would not need to contact her physician. However, based on Julie's age being older than 45 years and that she was not accustomed to vigorous activity, Maria recommended that she start with a moderate-intensity program. Julie and Maria both signed the PAR-Q+ form for the record. Maria also said that if Julie had answered "yes" to any of the follow-up questions she would then have to complete the ePARmed-X+ survey online or see her physician.

Demonstration Case Study 1.2

PAR-Q+

James is a 45-year-old man who is slightly overweight. He visits his physician once a year to get his annual physical. James noticed his blood pressure had been going up over the last several years. At his last physical exam his blood pressure was 150/94 mm Hg and his physician decided to put him on medication for high blood pressure. Since then, his blood pressure has been consistently around 126/84 mm Hg. James realizes that he is at risk for coronary artery disease (CAD) and wants to do something about it. He joins the local YMCA and meets with an exercise physiologist named Frances about getting started on an exercise program.

Frances starts by asking James a few questions and having him complete the PAR-Q+. He answers "yes" to question 1 because his doctor said he has high blood pressure and "no" to questions 2 to 7. Since he answered "yes" to at least one question, Frances had him complete the 10 questions on pages 2 and 3. James answered "no" to all questions except number 4 about high blood pressure. Therefore, he had to answer the two follow-up questions (4a and 4b) for number 4. Since he has been controlling his blood pressure (question 4a) and his blood pressure is lower than 160/90 mm Hg (question 4b), he answered "no" to both questions. Frances then directed him to page 4, which indicated that since he answered "no" to all of the 10 questions and/or subquestions, he is ready to become more physically active. They both signed the form for his records and Frances began to prescribe his exercise program.

Demonstration Case Study 1.3

ACSM Preparticipation Screening Algorithm

Michelle is a 47-year-old woman who has been walking 30 minutes per day, five days per week, for the last three years. She recently decided that she would like to begin running and eventually run a 5K race. After hearing about a local running club she decided to join and train with a group for a 5K race.

The trainer for the running group is LeBron, who is an ACSM Certified Exercise Physiologist® (EP-C). As part of good practice, he requires all new runners be screened. When Michelle meets with LeBron he asks her to complete a form about current activity levels; medical conditions; and potential signs or symptoms of cardiovascular, metabolic, or renal diseases. Michelle indicates that although she has no medical conditions she sometimes has a burning sensation in her chest when she walks at fast paces. LeBron recognizes this as a sign or symptom of disease. Using the ACSM Preparticipation Screening Algorithm, LeBron Instructs Michelle to discontinue her current exercise program until she obtains medical clearance from her physician. LeBron explains to Michelle that whenever a patient or client is symptomatic for a cardiovascular, metabolic, or renal disease he or she must seek medical clearance before beginning or continuing an exercise program.

Demonstration Case Study 1.4

ACSM Preparticipation Screening Algorithm

Enrique is an apparently healthy 36-year-old man who wants to complete a 150-mile hike over hilly terrain with some friends. The problem is he has not exercised regularly since attending college. He is a computer programmer and spends most of his time at work and home sitting. He knows that if he is going to be able to complete the hike he will have to start getting into shape, so he makes an appointment to meet with an ACSM EP-C named Tom. Enrique tells Tom he would like to start an exercise program of brisk walking up the steep hill outside of town. He believes this will get him prepared to do the hike with his friends.

Tom has Enrique complete a form about current activity levels, medical conditions, and potential signs or symptoms for cardiovascular, metabolic, or renal diseases. It is clear to Tom that Enrique is generally healthy but does not currently exercise. Using the ACSM Preparticipation Screening Algorithm, Tom explains that because Enrique has no known chronic diseases and no signs or symptoms of those chronic diseases he does not need medical clearance to begin exercising. However, because he has not been exercising regularly it is necessary for him to begin at a moderate intensity. Therefore, he should not start with walking up the steep hill outside of town, but rather walk briskly on flatter ground until he develops better aerobic fitness and exercise tolerance. After that, he can gradually work in some uphill walking over time and be ready for the hike with his friends next summer.

Student Case Study 1.1

PAR-Q+

Paul is a 66-year-old, recently retired man who averaged 60-hour work weeks over 30 years in a sedentary desk job. Despite his lack of physical activity he is generally healthy. Now that he has more free time he wants to begin an exercise program. He goes to a fitness facility and inquires about membership options. Per facility policy, all new members are required to complete the PAR-Q+. He is given the first page of the PAR-Q+ and he answers "no" to all seven questions. What should be recommended to Paul as the next steps based on these results?

1. Does he need to complete pages 2 and 3 of the PAR-Q+. Why or why not?
2. Does he need to complete the ePARmed-X+. Why or why not?
3. Can he begin the exercise program? Why or why not?
4. Should Paul perform moderate or vigorous exercise? Why?

Student Case Study 1.2

PAR-Q+

Kathleen is a 49-year-old woman who recently had breast cancer. She previously had a lumpectomy and completed chemotherapy. She is currently in remission and beginning to feel stronger, so she wants to begin an exercise program. She heard that exercise could improve her prognosis. The rest of her health is very good.

Based on her physician's recommendation Kathleen visits a hospital-based fitness center where you work. She joins the fitness center as a member and goes to an orientation. As part of the orientation she completes the PAR-Q+. On the first page she marks "no" to all questions except number 4, which she marks "yes" and lists "breast cancer." What should be recommended to Kathleen as the next steps based on these results?

1. Does she need to complete pages 2 and 3 of the PAR-Q+. Why or why not?
2. Does she need to complete the ePARmed-X+. Why or why not?
3. Can she begin the exercise program? Why or why not?

4. Should Kathleen perform moderate or vigorous exercise? Why?

Student Case Study 1.3

Lorenzo is a 36-year-old male portfolio manager for an investment firm that just opened an on-site fitness center for the employees. One of the staff exercise physiologists must screen all participants before they begin exercising in the new facility. Each new member must answer a set of questions that are used in the ACSM Preparticipation Screening Algorithm. Lorenzo says he has been exercising regularly (30 minutes of vigorous running, three times per week) for several years, has no known chronic diseases, and has no signs or symptoms of chronic disease. Based on this information, what should be recommended to Lorenzo before he can begin exercising in the new facility?

1. Should he get medical clearance before beginning? Why or why not?
2. Should he perform moderate or vigorous exercise? Why?
3. Should he get medical clearance before progressing to higher intensities? Why or why not?

Student Case Study 1.4

Hillary is a 63-year-old woman who comes to a community recreation center to begin exercising. She is very interested in a beginning yoga class but would also like to try some of the cardio equipment. She meets with an exercise physiologist for an orientation session that also includes a preparticipation health screening using the ACSM algorithm. In the conversation with Hillary it is determined that she has no signs or symptoms of chronic disease. However, she did have a minor heart attack two years ago. Despite a recommendation to start exercising regularly after her heart attack, she delayed making that commitment until now. Hillary had an appointment with her physician last week and she was again cleared for and advised to start exercising. This gave her the motivation to start an exercise program. As a result of this discussion with Hillary what should be recommended to her before starting the program?

1. Should she get medical clearance before beginning? Why or why not?
2. Should she perform moderate or vigorous exercise? Why?
3. Should she get medical clearance before progressing to higher intensities? Why or why not?

REFERENCES

1. American College of Sports Medicine. *ACSM's Guidelines for Exercise Testing and Prescription*, 11th edition. Philadelphia, PA: Wolters Kluwer Health, 2022.

2. Bredin SS, Gledhill N, Jamnik VK, Warburton DE. PAR-Q+ and ePARmed-X+: new risk stratification and physical activity clearance strategy for physicians and patients alike. *Can Fam Physician* 59(3): 273–277, 2013.

3. American College of Sports Medicine, 2022.

4. Bredin, Gledhill, Jamnik, and Warburton, 2013.

5. Bredin, Gledhill, Jamnik, and Warburton, 2013.

6. American College of Sports Medicine, 2022.

CHAPTER 2

Evaluation Before Exercise Prescription

INTRODUCTION

ONCE IT IS determined that someone is healthy enough to exercise safely, it is beneficial to obtain additional information on the risk factors for cardiovascular disease. Apparently healthy individuals in the health fitness setting do not require as much evaluation as those with chronic diseases. In an ideal situation it would be helpful to appraise the eight major risk factors. Half of these can be assessed by asking a few basic questions. Getting height, weight, and blood pressure measures provides information on two more. A simple blood test can determine the rest.

To complete the case studies in this chapter, students must learn the risk factors for atherosclerotic cardiovascular disease and the criteria for each. In the case studies in this chapter, it is important to extract the information needed to determine the risk factor status and disregard information that is not relevant. By getting an accurate count of the risk factors, exercise physiologists can help clients develop lifestyle goals and effective exercise prescriptions.

The purpose of this chapter is to teach students how to evaluate a client's risk profile. On completion of the case studies students will be able to:

1. Evaluate the following risk factors:
    a. Age
    b. Family history
    c. Cigarette smoking
    d. Physical activity
    e. Obesity
    f. Hypertension
    g. Dyslipidemia
    h. Diabetes
2. Define a negative risk factor
3. Determine risk factor count
4. Use risk factor status to make lifestyle recommendation

RISK FACTORS FOR ATHEROSCLEROTIC CARDIOVASCULAR DISEASE

Eight major risk factors have been recognized for atherosclerotic cardiovascular disease (CVD). These have been identified over the years and modified accordingly. There has been good consensus on which factors should be included. There is less consensus on the actual cutoffs that define each risk factor. For example, the cutoff for high systolic blood pressure is equal to or greater than 130 mm Hg. Some publications may have a slightly different number. Therefore, it is important to learn the criteria for the specific certification being pursued. In these case studies the standards recognized by the American College of Sports Medicine (ACSM) will be used to prepare for the Certified Exercise Physiologist® (EP-C) certification.[1]

Some risk factors are controllable and some are not. The first risk factor is age. Aging is a reality for all, and as people age their risk for atherosclerotic CVD increases. Therefore, men 45 years of age and older and women 55 years of age and older are considered to have a risk factor due to age.

Another uncontrollable risk factor is genetics, which is categorized as family history for CVD. When considering family history, data on only first-degree biological relatives should be used. First-degree relatives are defined as those who share 50% of the genes, such as parents, full siblings, and children. When determining the family history risk factor, exercise professionals should consider first-degree relatives who have died from CVD or had a myocardial infarction or coronary revascularization. The age cutoffs for these events are before 55 years old for male first-degree relatives and before 65 years old for female first-degree relatives.

One major risk factor that can be controlled is cigarette smoking. Current smokers have a higher risk for CVD, and the risk remains for six months after quitting. Non-smokers who are habitually exposed to second-hand smoke from other smokers are also at a higher risk.

Another CVD risk factor that is clearly controllable is physical inactivity. The general guideline for regular physical activity is participating in at least moderate-intensity physical activity for at least 75 minutes per week. Individuals who do not meet the afore-mentioned guidelines for regular physical would have the physical inactivity risk factor.

Excess body fat is another controllable risk factor for CVD. There are many methods to define body composition and the criteria for the excess body fat risk factor do not directly take into account the amount of body fat. They are the body mass index (BMI) and waist girth. The BMI is the person's weight in kilograms divided by the person's height in meters squared. If the BMI is equal to or greater than 30 kg/m^2 the person is considered at higher risk due to obesity. As BMI does not discriminate between muscle and fat, people with large muscle masses may erroneously be classified as obese. Therefore some exercise professionals prefer to use waist girth, which is an assessment of central adiposity. It is important that the measurements be taken in the correct place on the waist. For waist circumference to be a valid assessment of body composition, the circumference should be taken just below the lowest rib. For men, a measurement greater than 40 inches and for women, greater than 35 inches would be considered a higher risk for CVD. It is possible that someone with a BMI less than 30 kg/m² could have excess fat in the waist area and a waist circumference greater than the cutoff. Meeting the criterion for one test is sufficient to classify it as a positive risk factor.

A risk factor over which people have some control is hypertension. Blood pressure has two numbers: systolic pressure, which is the pressure the blood exerts against the blood vessel walls when the heart contracts, and diastolic pressure, which is the pressure the blood exerts against the blood vessel walls when the heart is at rest. Both systolic and diastolic blood pressures are important for health, and if either one is elevated there is an increased risk for CVD. The cutoffs for the hypertension risk factor is greater than or equal to 130 mm Hg for systolic blood pressure and 80 mm Hg for diastolic blood pressure. Only one of the pressures has to be above normal limits to count hypertension as a CVD risk factor. Many people take medication to lower their blood pressures and even though their pressures may be lower than the cutoffs, they still have the CVD risk because their pressures are too high without the medications.

Dyslipidemia is a risk factor that requires a blood test. As low-density lipoprotein cholesterol (LDL-C), in excessive amounts, is unhealthy and higher levels of high-density lipoprotein cholesterol (HDL-C) are healthy, it is best to get both numbers if possible. Sometimes only the total serum cholesterol is available. Because a higher concentration of LDL-C in the blood is associated with higher CVD risk, the cutoff for higher risk is 130 mg/dL. Because the HDL-C is a scavenger lipoprotein cholesterol, working in reverse of lipid transport, the cutoff is lower than 40 mg/dL for men and lower than 50 mg/dl for women. If the fractions are not available then the cutoff for total serum cholesterol is greater than or equal to 200 mg/dL. Additionally, all individuals who are on lipid-lowering medication would have this risk factor.

Blood glucose levels are also important for determining CVD risk because of the relationship between CVD and diabetes. The cutoff for plasma glucose levels which indicates an increased risk for CVD depends on the blood test used. Fasting plasma glucose levels greater than or equal to 100 mg/dL or two-hour plasma values of greater than or equal to 140 mg/dL from an oral glucose tolerance test would indicate higher risk for CVD. Because glucose levels can fluctuate greatly over short periods of time, a more stable test, of the glycolated hemoglobin value (HbA1C), can also be used. In this test an HbA1C value greater than or equal to 5.7% would indicate diabetes and a higher risk for CVD.

NEGATIVE RISK FACTOR FOR ATHEROSCLEROTIC CARDIOVASCULAR DISEASE

The previously discussed risk factors are positive risk factors because they indicate a higher risk for CVD. More recently, a high HDL-C level was determined to have protective value against CVD and is called a negative risk factor. The cutoff for HDL-C as a negative risk factor is greater than 60 mg/dL. Therefore, an HDL-C of less than 40 mg/dL is a positive risk factor and HDL-C of greater than 60 mg/dL is a negative risk factor. At this time, HDL-C is the only negative risk factor. Previously, all risk factors were considered bad for health, but now, a positive risk factor is bad and negative risk factor is good.

DETERMINING OVERALL RISK FACTOR STATUS

When working with a client, to get an idea of the overall risk for CVD, the negative risk factor (if it exists) is subtracted from the total number of positive risk factors. If a risk factor cannot be assessed, then it should be assumed that it is a risk factor. For example, if blood test data are not available and dyslipidemia and blood glucose cannot be assessed, then they both would be considered positive risk factors. Additionally, the negative risk factor (HDL-C) could not be considered. Likewise, if a client was adopted and does not know the biological family's health history then family history would be considered a positive risk factor. Although it is an arbitrary number, the sum of the positive risk factors minus the negative risk factor can provide a value of the overall risk for CVD.

APPLICATIONS FOR RISK FACTOR IDENTIFICATION

Clearly, identifying the factors that make someone more prone to experience a cardiovascular event is advantageous when talking with clients about lifestyle changes. Most cutoffs that are indicated as risk factors are areas that can be addressed. Obviously age and family history are not modifiable. Other risk factors can be improved by exercise and nutrition, as well as smoking cessation. Future chapters will focus on the development of exercise prescriptions to help reduce the risk for atherosclerotic CVD.

Demonstration Case Study 2.1

Risk factor profile

Josh is a male freshman college student who lives at home with his parents. He goes to the university rec center to get information and continue his exercise program. Lisa is an exercise physiologist and meets with Josh to go over his CVD risk profile. She asks Josh a few questions and finds out he is 18 years old. He has never smoked cigarettes but his father is a lifetime smoker and Josh has been exposed to his second-hand smoke since birth. Josh has exercised most of his life, as he was a football player through high school. He has lifted weights religiously and after graduating from high school has been running 12 miles per week. Both of his parents are alive but his father recently had heart bypass surgery at the age of 51 years. This prompted Josh to learn more about his CVD risk. Lisa measured Josh's weight and height and found he was 209 pounds and 74 inches tall. She took his blood pressure, which was 128/82 mm Hg and his resting heart rate was 70 beats per minute.

Recently Josh went to a health fair where they were offering free blood tests LDL-C and HDL-C. His results were LDL-C = 115 mg/dL, HDL-C = 62 mg/dL, and fasting plasma glucose = 99 mg/dL. He provided this information to Lisa so she could do a complete analysis of his risk factors.

Lisa evaluated the following risk factors:

Age—No. He is under 45 years old.

Family history—Yes. His father had coronary revascularization before the age of 55 years.

Cigarette smoking—Yes. Although Josh does not smoke he is and has been exposed to his father's second-hand smoke.

Physical inactivity—No. Josh has been running and lifting weights regularly.

Body mass index—No. Lisa calculates Josh's BMI by dividing his weight of 209 pounds by 2.2 to get 95.0 kilograms. Then she converts his height of 74 inches to meters by multiplying by .0254 and gets 1.9 meters. The height is then squared to get 3.6 meters squared. The BMI equals weight divided by his height in meters squared, so 95.0/3.6 = 26.4. Since the BMI is less than 30 kg/m² it is not a risk factor.

Blood pressure—Yes. His systolic pressure of 128 is under 140 mm Hg but his diastolic of 82 is over 80 mm Hg.

Lipids—No. His LDL-C of 115 is under 130 mg/dL and his HDL-C of 62 is over 40 mg/dL.

Blood glucose—No. Josh's fasting plasma glucose of 99 is under 126 mg/dL.

Negative risk factor—Yes. Because Josh's HDL-C of 62 is over 60 mg/dL this is considered a negative risk factor.

Based on the foregoing data, Lisa found Josh to have three positive CVD risk factors and one negative risk factor. Therefore, his number of risk factors for CVD is two. Lisa explains to Josh that this is a pretty good profile. Some risk factors cannot be controlled, such as his father's heart health. One way to improve his risk profile is to move from his parent's house so he will not be exposed to second-hand smoke. Also eating a healthier diet can help to lower his diastolic blood pressure.

Demonstration Case Study 2.2

Risk factor profile

Harriet is a 50-year-old woman who recently went to her physician, Dr. Smith, for a physical exam for the first time in 10 years. Dr. Smith was concerned about some of her tests and wrote an order for her to have an exercise stress test. Because she had not exercised in decades she did not tolerate the stress test very well, achieving only 6 METS but at least the test was negative for CVD. Dr. Smith recommended she join a reputable fitness center and slowly begin an exercise program to reduce her CVD risk factor profile.

When Harriet went to her orientation with Bill, the head exercise physiologist, he asked her several questions to determine her CVD risk. Fortunately, she had the reports from her physical exam and blood tests. Looking over the blood tests, Bill noticed the following: LDL-C = 158 mg/dL, HDL-C = 52 mg/dL, and fasting plasma glucose = 108 mg/dL. He then measured her height, weight, and blood pressure. She was 62 inches tall and weighed 182 pounds. Her blood pressure was 128/78 mm Hg. Bill then asked a few questions and found out she had never smoked cigarettes or lived with anyone who did. Her biological parents were still living and healthy but her mother's second husband died of a sudden heart attack at the age of 70. She also had a half-brother who died of a heart attack. He was only 51 years old. Bill asked if she was taking any medications and she said that since her physical exam she started taking a drug to lower her blood pressure.

After reviewing the information he received Bill evaluated the following risk factors:

Age—No. She is a woman under the age of 55 years.

Family history—No. Her biological parents are still healthy. Her mother had no cardiovascular events before the age of 65 years and her father had none before 55 years. Although her half-brother did have a fatal cardiovascular event before the age of 55 years it is not a family history risk factor because he is not a first-degree relative, defined as one who shares 50% of her genes. Only full siblings would count.

Cigarette smoking—No. Harriet never smoked.

Physical activity—Yes. She has not exercised regularly in decades.

BMI—Yes. Bill calculated Harriet's BMI by converting her weight to kilograms, 182 pounds/2.2 = 82.7 kg. Then he converted her height into meters, 62 inches × .0254 = 1.6 m and squared it to get 2.6 m^2. Using these conversions Bill calculated her BMI = 82.7/2.6 = 31.8 kg/m^2. Because her BMI is over 30 it is a positive risk factor.

Blood pressure—Yes. Although Bill took Harriet's blood pressure and it was under 130 mm Hg systolic and 80 mm Hg diastolic, she is currently taking medication to lower it. Therefore, hypertension is a risk factor for Harriet.

Lipids—Yes. Because her LDL-C is over 130 mg/dL this is a risk factor. Even though her HDL-C is over the recommended 50 mg/dL it takes only one of these two criteria to make it a positive risk factor.

Blood glucose—Yes. Her fasting plasma glucose is over 100 mg/dL.

Negative risk factor—No. Her HDL-C is not 60 mg/dL or higher, so this negative risk factor does not apply.

Using the information Bill obtained from Harriet, he determined she has five positive CVD risk factors and no negative risk factors. Therefore, Harriet has a total of five risk factors. At the end of the meeting Bill tells Harriet that she has a significant risk of future heart disease but she does have some control. Starting a regular exercise program at the fitness center would be a good start. After exercising regularly that risk factor would be removed. Bill also explains that regular exercise has benefits in controlling the other risk factors that she has, such as obesity, high blood pressure, high blood glucose and high blood cholesterol level. Bill says Harriet needs to make her diet healthier and that diet combined with exercise will help her lose weight. The exercise and resulting weight loss will also help her lower her blood glucose, blood pressure and blood cholesterol levels.

Student Case Study 2.1

Risk factor profile

Kenny is a lead guitarist in a local country band. He is living a pretty hard life, playing in local bars, staying up late every night, smoking cigarettes, and drinking beer. He generally sleeps in late and then has no time for planned physical activity. At the young age of 25 years old his body is beginning to feel the effects of his lifestyle. Then a month ago his 56-year-old father had a nonfatal heart attack. Although his mother is very healthy at 55 years old, his father's heart attack scared Kenny so he decided to get a physical from his physician and make some lifestyle changes. As part of his physical exam it was found that Kenny is 6 feet 3 inches tall and weighs 239 pounds. His blood pressure is 130/86 mm Hg. His blood test revealed his LDL-C = 125 mg/dL, HDL-C = 28 mg/dL, and fasting plasma glucose = 110 mg/dL.

1. What are the positive risk factors for CVD?
2. Why is each risk factor in question 1 qualified as a positive risk factor?
3. What are the negative risk factors for CVD?
4. Why is each risk factor in question 3 qualified as a negative risk factor?
5. Which risk factors does the client not have?
6. Why is each risk factor in question 5 not qualified as a risk factor?
7. How many CVD risk factors does the client have?
8. What lifestyle changes would you recommend? Why?

Student Case Study 2.2

Risk factor profile

Amanda is a 36-year-old mother of three children. Since her third pregnancy she has continued to gain weight and currently weighs 165 pounds, with a height of 61 inches. She visits her physician annually for a check-up. She currently has the following blood lipid levels: HDL-C = 42 mg/dL, LDL-C = 122 mg/dL, and fasting gluscose = 107 mg/dL. She is on a lipid-lowering drug because high cholesterol runs in her family. Both of her parents have high cholesterol but are otherwise in good health. Her blood pressure is 100/68 mm Hg. Amanda quit smoking before her first pregnancy 11 years ago and currently lives in a smoke-free environment. After her first pregnancy she started doing a spinning class three days per week and continues it to this day.

1. What are the positive risk factors for CVD?
2. Why is each risk factor in question 1 qualified as a positive risk factor?
3. What are the negative risk factors for CVD?
4. Why is each risk factor in question 3 qualified as a negative risk factor?
5. Which risk factors does the client not have?
6. Why is each risk factor in question 5 not qualified as a risk factor?
7. How many CVD risk factors does the client have?
8. What lifestyle changes would you recommend? Why?

Student Case Study 2.3

Risk factor profile

Brian is a 52-year-old man who has enjoyed physical activity all of his life. He likes to downhill ski, kayak, and hike for recreation and runs, bikes, and lifts weights to stay in shape for these hobbies by exercising at least 45 minutes at least five days per week. He was raised in a very health-conscious family and his parents, who are in their 70s, and three siblings in their 50s are all in excellent health. He has always tried to eat a healthy diet and never used tobacco or other drugs. He watches his weight but because he is quite muscular does not pay attention to the BMI. Instead, he watches his waist circumference, which measures 79 cm. He has an annual check-up with his physician every year. His last lab test results were: LDL-C = 101 mg/dL, HDL-C = 62 mg/dL, and fasting glucose = 90 mg/dL. His last blood pressure reading was 114/70 mm Hg.

1. What are the positive risk factors for CVD?
2. Why is each risk factor in question 1 qualified as a positive risk factor?
3. What are the negative risk factors for CVD?
4. Why is each risk factor in question 3 qualified as a negative risk factor?
5. Which risk factors does the client not have?
6. Why is each risk factor in question 5 not qualified as a risk factor?
7. How many CVD risk factors does the client have?
8. What lifestyle changes would you recommend? Why?

Naomi is a 49-year-old woman. Ten weeks ago she made the decision to start living healthier. She started by giving up smoking and that has gone well for her so far. At the same time she started a daily walking program that she feels cuts her craving to smoke. She also began to eat a healthier diet by reducing fat and eating more fresh fruits and vegetables. In ten weeks she has lost 20 pounds and now weighs 151 pounds on her 5 foot 4 inch frame. Every week at the grocery store she uses the free do-it-yourself blood pressure monitor and is happy that her blood pressure is down to 126/78 mm Hg from 136/90 mm Hg. Feeling that she is making good progress, she has a blood test done. Her report indicated the following: LDL-C = 92 mg/dL, HDL-C = 46 mg/dL, and fasting glucose = 103 mg/dL. Naomi believes these numbers are pretty good and will help her avoid the fate of her older brother, who had a major heart attack at the age of 52 years, but decides to ask, an exercise physiologist she knows, what he thinks.

1. What are the positive risk factors for CVD?
2. Why is each risk factor in question 1 qualified as a positive risk factor?
3. What are the negative risk factors for CVD?
4. Why is each risk factor in question 3 qualified as a negative risk factor?
5. Which risk factors does the client not have?
6. Why is each risk factor in question 5 not qualified as a risk factor?
7. How many CVD risk factors does the client have?
8. What lifestyle changes would you recommend? Why?

REFERENCE

1. American College of Sports Medicine. *ACSM's Guidelines for Exercise Testing and Prescription*, 11th edition. Philadelphia, PA: Wolters Kluwer Health, 2022.

CHAPTER 3

Physical Fitness Testing and Interpretation

INTRODUCTION

IN THE FIRST two chapters, the health status information of the client was considered. This chapter will consider the fitness status of an apparently healthy client. To write an effective exercise prescription, exercise physiologists need to understand the current fitness level of their clients by testing some of the components of fitness. The procedures for conducting fitness tests are very precise, and students should learn proper testing techniques in a laboratory class. This chapter will focus on the interpretations of selected fitness tests and how to classify or categorize the results as percentiles or categories.

The case studies presented will challenge students to make computations and evaluate the results. Many different fitness tests are available and those chosen will depend on the equipment available, time, expertise, cost, and space. The examples in this chapter will emphasize some of the more commonly used protocols. Students must familiarize themselves with the equations in order to complete the case studies.

The purpose of this chapter is to teach students how to calculate and interpret the data obtained from the fitness tests. On completion of the case studies, students will be able to:

1. Determine the risk classification for the body mass index (BMI)
2. Use circumference measurements to determine risk category
3. Calculate percent body fat from skinfold measurements and determine fitness percentile
4. Determine when to stop an exercise test to maintain safety standards
5. Estimate maximal oxygen consumption ($\dot{V}O_{2max}$) from field tests for cardiorespiratory fitness and classify fitness level
6. Categorize fitness level for grip strength
7. Determine fitness category for both upper body strength (bench press) and lower body strength (leg press)
8. Utilize push-up test data to find muscular endurance fitness category
9. Classify flexibility status using goniometer data
10. Use countermovement vertical jump data to determine muscular power category

FITNESS TESTING BASICS

The purposes of fitness testing include obtaining baseline data to determine fitness status (by comparing results with normative data) and to write good exercise prescriptions. Follow-up testing is used to monitor progress and evaluate the effectiveness of the exercise prescription. Appropriate modifications of the exercise program are frequently made as a result of follow-up testing. When clients see improvements in their fitness tests it helps to increase their motivation to continue exercising.

The most important considerations when conducting fitness tests are safety, validity, and reliability. Safety begins with an informed consent and a pre-participation health screening discussed in Chapter 1. A pre-exercise evaluation of medical history and risk factors for cardiovascular disease (CVD) should follow to develop a better understanding of the client's condition (discussed in Chapter 2).

To improve validity and reliability, all equipment must be examined to make sure it is in good working order and calibrated. Ideally the testing order should begin with resting measures and proceed from least intense to most intense activities. If a heart rate–dependent test is to be performed, it needs to be conducted first, as the heart rate may remain elevated after an exercise test and thereby diminish the reliability of the heart rate–dependent test. The same muscle groups should not be repeatedly worked, and adequate recovery should be provided between tests. The test environment should be comfortable and relaxed. All testing sessions should be conducted in a consistent manner so accurate comparisons can be made over time.

TYPES OF FITNESS TESTS

There are many different fitness tests for the various components of fitness. Depending on the goals of the client, different tests can be chosen. Most exercise prescriptions for health should include resting values, body composition, cardiorespiratory fitness, muscular fitness, and flexibility.

Resting values. Typical resting values that are collected include resting heart rate and resting blood pressure. Lower resting heart rates are found with better cardiorespiratory fitness and they are used in some calculations such as the heart rate reserve method for heart rate prescriptions. There are no normative data for resting heart rate. Blood pressure fluctuates widely over the day depending on stress and activity. Resting blood pressure is one of the risk factors for CVD discussed in Chapter 2.

Body composition. Poor body composition is a CVD risk factor. There are several ways to compute body composition. For risk factor status, the BMI is commonly used. To determine BMI, height and weight must be measured as part of the testing. Because the BMI does not differentiate between fat weight and muscle weight (or other nonfat weight), some prefer to use waist circumference. Although not the most accurate for body composition, many people have excess fat deposited in the waist area, and waist circumference will take this into consideration. The results of the BMI can be used to classify clients as underweight, normal, overweight, or in one of three classes of obesity. The cutoff for CVD risk is 30. Waist circumference can be used to categorize clients' risk, ranging from very low to very high. If both values are obtained they can be combined to get a better measure of risk for disease.

A better way to assess body composition is by conducting a skinfold assessment, which provides a good estimation of the amount of body fat. There are many protocols available that use various numbers of the approximately nine commonly measured skinfold sites. Using the skinfold measurements for the specific protocol, the body density can be calculated. The body density is then converted mathematically to percent body fat. The recommended percent of body fat is not widely agreed on. However, charts are available to classify individuals in percentiles and categorize them from very lean to very poor. To save time, the protocol should be determined in advance and only the specific skinfold sites needed should be measured.

Cardiorespiratory fitness. Cardiorespiratory fitness is often quantified by measuring $\dot{V}O_{2max}$. The best method for determining $\dot{V}O_{2max}$ is to conduct a maximal graded exercise test and collect expired gases using a metabolic cart. However, the test is costly and most facilities do not have access to a metabolic cart. Therefore the $\dot{V}O_{2max}$ is usually estimated. The estimation of $\dot{V}O_{2max}$ can be done by performing a maximal graded exercise test without expired gas collection, a submaximal graded exercise test, or a field test. The type of exercise is usually walking or running but cycling (leg ergometer) and stepping can also be used. Formulas are available to estimate $\dot{V}O_{2max}$ based on test performance. If a maximal graded exercise test is used, the protocol has metabolic equivalents for each stage. If a submaximal graded exercise test is used the data must be extrapolated. Generally maximal workload is estimated by taking submaximal workloads and projecting them to an estimated maximal heart rate. This can be done because there is a direct linear relationship between workload and heart rate. Field tests have formulas based on time and distance covered. Other tests may not estimate $\dot{V}O_{2max}$ but categorize the performance based on other variables such as heart rate response.

The test used to determine $\dot{V}O_{2max}$ should be selected based on the accuracy of results expected and the time and equipment available. If $\dot{V}O_{2max}$ is determined directly or estimated the results can be compared to normative data based on age and sex. Percentile score and category from very poor to superior can be found.

Muscular fitness. The components of muscular fitness include strength, endurance, and power. Power is important for health but more important for athletic performance. When doing fitness testing for health, power is now recommended to be tested. Strength and endurance have always been considered important for health and daily living so these two components are commonly tested.

Determining maximal strength is challenging. If the one-repetition maximal (1-RM) is used the tester must estimate the maximal amount to be performed. Then it is trial and error. If the weight is lifted then more weight is added. If the weight is too much, then weight needs to be removed. With each attempt the person being tested becomes more fatigued and if the test takes too long the fatigue will negatively affect the accuracy of the test. Clearly the beginning weight is easier to predict in post-testing than for the initial test.

An option for the 1-RM is to use a dynamometer. Fatigue is not as much of an issue because the person being tested does a maximal contraction and the instrument records the amount of force generated. However, because the contraction moves through a very limited range of motion it is closer to an isometric contraction than a concentric contraction.

Another issue with muscle testing in general is there are many joints in the human body in which muscles contract and they all can have different levels of strength. The question is which joints or muscle groups to test. The most common tests for the 1-RM are bench press and leg press. For dynamometers the most common is grip strength.

For muscular endurance the muscle group to test must be identified as well. The most commonly used muscular endurance tests are push-ups and sit-ups. The American College of Sports Medicine (ACSM) recently announced that the sit-up test is not recommended, as the test may cause low back injuries. The push-up test will be used in the following case studies. It should be noted that there are several different push-up protocols, so it is important to follow the specific testing guidelines for the normative data that will be used.

The results of the muscle tests have categorical descriptions and/or percentiles based on age and sex. The performance for the grip strength the highest score of either hand and the number of push-ups successfully completed can be categorized from poor to excellent. The 1-RM can be rated as percentile using the weight pushed divided by body weight and also classified as very poor to superior.

TERMINATING A GRADED EXERCISE TEST

Graded exercise tests have a predetermined end point. For maximal tests the end point is when the person can no longer continue or volitional fatigue sets in. Usually the heart rate has maxed out, lactic acid has accumulated to intolerable levels, and oxygen consumption has leveled off. Submaximal tests are usually stopped when the client reaches 85% of the age-predicted maximal heart rate. Some submaximal tests end when a specific stage of the test is completed or simply after a specific time of exercise.

The previously described criteria are assuming that the person being tested is healthy enough to complete the test. Despite using health screenings before testing individuals there is always a chance the screening was not 100% accurate. In these cases it is important for the exercise physiologist to know when to stop the test before the exerciser has any health complications!

Before attempting the case studies in this chapter the indications for stopping an exercise test must be learned. It is important to remember that these guidelines are for apparently healthy individuals and will differ from the guidelines for individuals with known or suspected disease. The latter guidelines apply to tests conducted for diagnostic purposes. As this chapter focuses on healthy people, any indication of disease must result in the termination of the test and a medical evaluation to determine if the individual is healthy enough to begin or continue an exercise program. In summary, some of the common reasons for stopping the test prematurely include pain in the chest, trouble breathing, leg cramps, change in skin color, dizziness, or abnormal heart rate or blood pressure responses.

Demonstration Case Study 3.1

Physical fitness testing and interpretation

Benjamin is a 36-year-old man who comes to the fitness center for fitness testing by the exercise physiologist Graham. The results of his tests are:

- height = 74 inches
- weight = 201 pounds
- chest skinfolds = 9 mm
- triceps skinfold = 11 mm
- thigh skinfold = 15 mm
- subscapular skinfold = 16 mm
- Cooper 12-minute walk/run test = 2150 meters
- right hand grip strength = 49 kg
- left hand grip strength = 46 kg
- push-ups = 19
- shoulder flexion = 169 degrees
- hip extention = 16 degrees
- hip flexion = 131 degrees

Graham uses these data to calculate Benjamin's fitness status for the BMI, percent body fat, cardiorespiratory fitness, muscular strength, muscular endurance, and flexibility.

First, he calculates the BMI.

$$BMI = \text{weight (kg)}/(\text{height (m)})^2$$

Weight = 201 pounds/2.2 kg/pound = 91.36 kg

Height = 74 inches × .0254 meter/inch = 1.88 meters

$$Height^2 = (1.88 \text{ meters})^2 = 3.53 \text{ meters}^2$$

$$BMI = 92.36 \text{ kg}/3.53 \text{ m}^2 = 26.16 \text{ kg/m}^2$$

Comparing this to the BMI standards Benjamin is overweight.

Next Graham calculates the percent body fat using the three-site formula, which is the sum of the chest, triceps, and subscapular skinfolds. The thigh skinfold is not needed in this calculation.

Sum of three skinfolds = 9 mm + 11 mm + 16 mm = 36 mm

Body density = 1.1125025 – 0.0013125 (sum of 3) + 0.0000055 (sum of 3)^2 – 0.000244 (age)

Body density = 1.1125025 – 0.0013125 (36) + 0.0000055 (36)^2 – 0.000244 (36)

Body density = 1.1125025 – 0.0013125 (36) + 0.0000055 (1296) – 0.000244 (36)

Body density = 1.1125025 – 0.047250 + 0.007128 – 0.0087840

Body density = 1.063597

Percent body fat = [(4.95/Db) – 4.50] × 100

Percent body fat = [(4.95/1.063597) – 4.50] × 100

Percent body fat = 15.40

Graham compares Benjamin's body fat with the norms for his age and finds he is between the 75th and 80th percentiles, which is good/excellent. Although his BMI indicates Benjamin is overweight, his percent body fat is healthy. This is an example of a person with good muscle mass, which increases his BMI but decreases his percent body fat. Because the BMI does not differentiate between fat weight and muscle weight, Graham tells Benjamin his body composition is fine.

Looking at the results of the Cooper 12-minute walk/run test, Graham calculates Benjamin's estimated $\dot{V}O_{2max}$ using the distance Benjamin covered as equal to 2,150 meters.

VO_{2max} (mL/kg-min) = [distance (m) – 504.9]/44.73

VO_{2max} (mL/kg-min) = [2150 – 504.9]/44.73

VO_{2max} (mL/kg-min) = 36.78

Comparing Benjamin's result with the normative chart (treadmill-based max oxygen consumption), Graham finds his cardiorespiratory fitness classification to be between the 25th and 30th percentiles. This percentile is considered poor.

Moving to muscle testing, Graham checks the strength test using the hand dynamometer scores. Graham takes the highest of the left- and right-hand scores.

49 kg right and 46 kg left for a high score of 49 kg

When comparing Benjamin's score with the normative charts, 49 kg is slightly over the 50th percentile. For muscular endurance, Graham takes the push-up test score of 19 push-ups and compares it to the normative data. Benjamin's muscular endurance is classified as good.

Finally, Graham checks the flexibility score. Benjamin's scores of 169 degrees for shoulder flexion is average, 16 degrees for hip extention is below average and 131 degrees for hip flexion is above average. Based on the results of the test battery, Graham notes that Benjamin is average in muscular strength, muscular endurance, and flexibility. He definitely needs to work on his aerobic fitness. Graham will take these into consideration when he writes Benjamin's exercise prescription.

Demonstration Case Study 3.2

Physical fitness testing and interpretation

Sofia is a 27-year-old woman who comes to the fitness center for fitness testing by the exercise physiologist Karen. The results of her tests are:

- height = 63 inches

- weight = 119 pounds
- chest skinfolds = 10 mm
- triceps skinfold = 13 mm
- thigh skinfold = 14 mm
- subscapular skinfold = 19 mm
- midaxillary skinfold = 16
- abdomen skinfold = 21
- suprailiac skinfold = 23
- right hand grip strength = 28 kg
- left hand grip strength = 27 kg
- push-ups = 15
- modified YMCA cycle ergometer test results:

Stage	Resistance (kg)	Worklad (kg m/min)	Heart Rate (beats per minute)
I	0.5	150	99
II	1.5	450	120
III	2.0	600	138

Karen uses these data to calculate her fitness status for the BMI, percent body fat, cardiorespiratory fitness, muscular strength, muscular endurance, and flexibility.

First, she calculates the BMI.

BMI = weight (kg)/(height (m))^2

Weight = 119 pounds/2.2 kg/pound = 54.10 kg

Height = 63 inches × .0254 meter/inch = 1.60 meters

Height^2 = (1.60 meters)^2 = 2.56 meters^2

BMI = 54.10 kg/2.56 m^2 = 21.13 kg/m^2

Comparing this to the BMI standards Sofia is normal weight.

Next Karen calculates the percent body fat using the seven-site formula, which is the sum of the chest, midaxillary, triceps, subscapular, abdomen, suprailiac, and thigh skinfolds.

Sum of seven skinfolds = 10 mm + 16 mm + 13 mm + 19 mm + 21 mm + 23 mm + 14 mm
= 116 mm

Body density = 1.097 – 0.00046971 (sum of 7) + 0.00000056 (sum of 7)^2 –
0.00012828 (age)

Body density = 1.097 – 0.00046971 (116) + 0.00000056 (116)^2 – 0.00012828 (27)

Body density = 1.097 – 0.00046971 (116) + 0.00000056 (13456) – 0.00012828 (27)

Body density = 1.097 – 0.05448636 + 0.00753536 – 0.00346356

Body density = 1.0458544

Percent body fat = [(4.95/Db) – 4.50] × 100

Percent body fat = [(4.95/1.0458544) – 4.50] × 100

Percent body fat = 23.30

Karen compares Sofia's body fat with the norms for her age and finds she is between the 40th and 45th percentiles, which is fair. Her BMI is normal.

Looking at the results of the modified YMCA cycle ergometer test, Karen calculates Sofia's estimated $\dot{V}O_{2max}$ by projecting the line determined by two submaximal data points to her estimated maximal heart rate. Per the protocol, Karen needs two heart rates 110 beats per minute or higher and the corresponding workloads. Looking back at the test data, stage I data were not used because the heart rate was under 110 beats per minute. Her stage I heart rate was 99 beats per minute, which is the reason the resistance was increased to 1.5 kg in stage II. The resistance for stage III is always 0.5 kg higher than for stage II. The test is terminated by protocol when the second heart rate of 110 beats per minute or higher is attained or if Sofia reaches 85% of her estimated maximal heart rate based on her age, which was (220 – 27) × .85 = 164 beats per minute.

Karen could draw a graph using the two sets of data points but she is proficient in algebra and knows that drawing a graph has more inherent errors. So she determines the formula for the line by first obtaining the slope, which equals the change in y (heart rate) over the change in x (workload).

Slope (m) = 138 – 120/600 – 450 = 0.12 (138–120)/(600–450)

The line formula is $y = mx + b$, where m is the slope and b is the y-intercept.

Using either one of the sets of points for x and y, then 138 = 0.12(600) + b.

Solving for b, 138 = 72 + b, which means b = 66.

Therefore the formula for the line is $y = 0.12x + 66$.

Since Karen expects Sonia would stop at her estimated maximal heart rate of 193 beats per minute if it was a maximal test, she substitutes 193 for y: 193 = 0.12x + 66.

Therefore 127 = 0.12x or x = 1058, which is the workload Karen would predict at maximal exercise. Karen then uses the maximal workload to compute the $\dot{V}O_{2max}$ using the metabolic equation for leg cycling. (This calculation will be covered in more detail in Chapter 5.)

VO_{2max} = (1.8 × maximal work rate)/body mass + 7

VO_{2max} = (1.8 × 1058/54.10) + 7

VO_{2max} = 35.20 + 7

VO_{2max} = 42.20 mL/kg-min

Comparing Sofia's result with the normative chart for cycle ergometery, Karen finds her cardiorespiratory fitness classification to be between the 85th and 90th percentiles. This percentile is considered excellent.

Moving to muscle testing, Karen checks the strength test using the hand dynamometer scores. Karen takes the highest of the left- and right-hand scores.

28 kg for the right and 27 kg for the left = 28 kg

When comparing Sofia's score with the normative charts, 28 kg is classified as the 50th percentile. For muscular endurance Karen uses the push-up test score of 15 push-ups and compares it to the normative data. Sofia's muscular endurance is classified as good.

Based on the results of the test battery Karen notes that Sofia is in the 50th percentile in muscular strength and muscular endurance is good. Her body composition is at the higher end of normal and her cardiorespiratory fitness is excellent. Overall she is in good shape but has more to benefit from a regularly scheduled exercise program.

Demonstration Case Study 3.3

Physical fitness testing and interpretation

Layne is an exercise physiologist at a health and fitness center who is about to conduct a submaximal graded exercise test on a treadmill. Her client is Billy Joe, who has completed the screening process and found to be healthy and able to perform the test. His pre-test information is:

- 42 years old
- resting heart rate = 74 beats per minute
- resting blood pressure = 136/88 mm Hg

Because Layne is conducting a submaximu test, she first estimates Billy Joe's max heart rate by taking 220 minus his age (220 − 42 = 178) to get 178 beats per minute. Then she takes 85% of his estimated max heart rate (178 × 0.85 = 151) and gets 151 beats per minute as the point where she will stop the test. She begins the test and it progresses as follows:

Stage	Minute of Test	Heart Rate (beats per minute)	Blood Pressure (mm Hg)	Other
I	1	92		
I	2	97		
I	3	97	164/90	
II	4	110		
II	5	117		
II	6	118	192/98	
III	7	130		
III	8	136		
III	9	136	228/114	Legs begin to get sore
IV	10	148	230/118	

In the 10th minute Layne stops the test because Billy Joe's diastolic blood pressure surpassed 115 mm Hg even though Billy Joe did not reach the predetermined stopping point for the submaximal test of the heart rate, reaching 151 beats per minute. She did not stop the test because of sore legs because that is a normal effect of walking on a treadmill, especially up a grade. Layne informs Billy Joe he needs to talk with his physician about his blood pressure before beginning an exercise program.

Demonstration Case Study 3.4

Physical fitness testing and interpretation

Regan wants to begin an aerobic exercise program and goes to the local health and fitness club. Ronnell, the exercise physiologist, has her complete the screening process and finds she is healthy and can do a maximal treadmill test. In the pre-test Ronnell records the following data about Regan:

- 53 years old
- resting heart rate = 76 beats per minute
- resting blood pressure = 118/80 mm Hg

Ronnell begins the test and obtains the following data:

Stage	Minute of Test	Heart Rate (beats per minute)	Blood Pressure (mm Hg)	Other
I	1	94		
I	2	96		
I	3	96	128/80	
II	4	112		
II	5	120		
II	6	122	138/82	
III	7	132	146/80	Pain in the chest area

He stops the test in the 7th minute. Since Regan is an apparently healthy woman she would not be expected to have chest pain. The cause and type of the chest pain must be medically determined before she can begin or continue an exercise program.

Student Case Study 3.1

Physical fitness testing and interpretation

Betty is a 52-year-old woman who comes to the fitness center for fitness testing. After screening for health she is tested. The results of her tests are:

- height = 68 inches

- weight = 105 pounds
- chest skinfolds = 7 mm
- triceps skinfold = 8 mm
- thigh skinfold = 12 mm
- suprailiac skinfold = 14 mm
- 1.5 mile walk/run test = 18 minutes and 20 seconds
- right hand grip strength = 24 kg
- left hand grip strength = 22 kg
- push-ups = 9
- counter movement vertical jump = 16 cm

Determine her fitness status.

1. Calculate her BMI.
2. Calculate her percent body fat.
3. Calculate her predicted $\dot{V}O_{2max}$.
4. Calculate her grip strength score.
5. Determine her BMI weight status.
6. Determine her percent body fat fitness category and percentile.
7. Determine her cardiovascular fitness classification and percentile.
8. Determine her fitness category for grip strength.
9. Determine her fitness category for push-ups.
10. Determine her fitness category for the vertical jump test.

Student Case Study 3.2

Physical fitness testing and interpretation

Adam completes a submaximal cycle ergometer test. His resting values were:

- 58 years old
- resting heart rate = 72 beats per minute
- resting blood pressure = 126/72 mm Hg

The test results were:

Stage	Minute of Test	Heart Rate (beats per minute)	Blood Pressure (mm Hg)	Other
I	1	98		
I	2	104		
I	3	106	138/74	
II	4	116		
II	5	118		
II	6	118	144/74	

Stage	Minute of Test	Heart Rate (beats per minute)	Blood Pressure (mm Hg)	Other
III	7	129		
III	8	135		
III	9	138	154/74	
IV	10	144		
IV	11	146	166/72	
IV	12	148	166/74	Beginning to breathe noticeably harder without wheezing

1. Determine the submaximal heart rate at which the test should be stopped if reached.
2. Determine which minute of the test it should be terminated and why.

Student Case Study 3.3

Physical fitness testing and interpretation

Brittany completes a max treadmill test. Her resting values were:

- 62 years old
- resting heart rate = 79 beats per minute
- resting blood pressure = 132/86 mm Hg

The test results were:

Stage	Minute of Test	Heart Rate (beats per minute)	Blood Pressure (mm Hg)	Other
I	1	100		
I	2	106		
I	3	106	152/86	
II	4	116		
II	5	124		
II	6	125	168/86	
III	7	134		
III	8	136		
III	9	136	150/84	Leg cramps
IV	10	148		
IV	11	154		
IV	12	156	152/86	Subject requests to stop

1. Determine the submaximal heart rate at which the test should be stopped if reached.
2. Determine which minute of the test it should be terminated and why.

Student Case Study 3.4

Physical fitness testing and interpretation

Vicki completes a maximal treadmill test. Her resting values were:

- 36 years old
- resting heart rate = 62 beats per minute
- resting blood pressure = 102/66 mm Hg

The test results were:

Stage	Minute of Test	Heart Rate	Blood Pressure	Other
I	1	90		
I	2	96		
I	3	96	122/66	
II	4	112		
II	5	124		
II	6	126	138/66	
III	7	144		
III	8	156		
III	9	156	146/62	
IV	10	176		Deep rhythmic breathing
IV	11	184		
IV	12	186	152/64	Subject requests to stop

1. Determine the submaximal heart rate at which the test should be stopped if reached if it was a submax test.
2. Determine which minute of the test it should be terminated and why.

CHAPTER 4

Clinical Exercise
Testing and Interpretation

INTRODUCTION

CERTIFIED EXERCISE PHYSIOLOGISTS are prepared to test the fitness of and prescribe exercise to healthy individuals or those with controlled diseases. Although they have limited contact with the clinical population or those with suspected ischemic heart disease, they still need to understand some of the clinical concepts of diagnostic exercise testing. For example, the ACSM Certified Exercise Physiologist® is prepared to work with apparently healthy individuals, but sometimes an apparently healthy individual is not actually healthy. The person may have had a diagnostic exercise that was negative for cardiovascular disease (CVD). However, it could have been a false-negative test and the person actually has CVD. Therefore, the certified exercise physiologist must be aware that all tests are not accurate and know how to support such clients. A working knowledge of these concepts helps prepare the certified exercise physiologist to better recognize abnormal exercise responses and ensure the safe and effective supervision of apparently healthy clients and those with controlled diseases during an exercise program. Moreover, this knowledge is useful when educating clients about their health and the need for regular exercise.

This chapter will not attempt to cover material about how a clinical exercise test is performed. Rather, it will include concepts of what is learned from the tests and how well the tests diagnose ischemic heart disease. In particular, the case studies will deal with the concepts of pre-test likelihood of ischemic heart disease, post-test prognosis, and the diagnostic value of clinical exercise testing.

The purpose of this chapter is to teach students how to evaluate the applications and effectiveness of clinical exercise testing. On completion of the case studies, students will be able to:

1. Determine the pre-test likelihood of ischemic heart disease
2. Ascertain the post-test prognosis of ischemic heart disease
3. Compute the effectiveness of maximal exercise testing for diagnosing ischemic heart disease including:
   a. Sensitivity
   b. Specificity

c. Positive predictive value

d. Negative predictive value

PRE-TEST LIKELIHOOD OF ISCHEMIC HEART DISEASE

In general, the likelihood that someone has ischemic heart disease before or without the results of a graded exercise test is dependent on age, sex, and the type of chest pain experienced, if any. Men and women of any age who do not experience any type of chest pain, or in other words are asymptomatic, have low or very low pre-test likelihoods of ischemic heart disease. The presence and the characteristics of the chest pain then determines whether the likelihood is intermediate or high.

Because certified exercise physiologists work with apparently healthy individuals anyone with chest pain would be referred for medical evaluation before exercise. These people would be screened out by the PAR-Q+ or the American College of Sports Medicine Pre-participation Screening Algorithm. Only after being cleared by a medical evaluation or possibly a negative graded exercise test would they be ready for an exercise prescription from a certified exercise physiologist.

Determining the pre-test likelihood of ischemic heart disease is as simple as using a table.[1] The more challenging part is determining the type of chest pain if it exists. The definitions of chest pain and how to use the chart should be reviewed before completing the case studies presented below.

POST-TEST PROGNOSIS FOR ISCHEMIC HEART DISEASE

After someone has a diagnostic graded exercise test there will be more and better information to determine the status of ischemic heart disease. The factors that are used for the post-test prognosis include the maximum metabolic equivalents (METs) attained in the graded exercise test, the presence and degree of angina, and the maximum ST segment deviation from baseline on the electrocardiograph during the test. This information is used in the Duke Nomogram.[2] By accurately connecting the data points in the nomogram, the five-year survival rate and the average annual mortality rate can be determined.

EFFECTIVENESS OF DIAGNOSTIC TESTING

Despite the best efforts of clinicians, the diagnostic results for a graded exercise test are not 100% accurate. Some people test positive for ischemic heart disease but do not have it. This is a false-positive test. Others may test negative but actually have ischemic heart disease. This would be a false-negative test. The goal is to have all tests be true positives, where all the people tested who have ischemic heart disease test positive, or true negatives, where all the people tested who do not have ischemic heart disease test negative.

To evaluate the effectiveness of diagnostic testing, the graded exercise test can be validated with additional, more accurate tests. Once the number of true-positive, true-negative, false-positive, and false-negative tests has been determined, the sensitivity, specificity, and predictive values of the testing can be calculated. The case studies provide an opportunity to practice making these calculations.

Demonstration Case Study 4.1

Clinical exercise testing and interpretation

LeRoy is a 68-year-old male who reports to the local hospital for a scheduled graded exercise test. He was referred for testing by his physician because he recently developed typical angina with exertion. He meets with Kaitlyn, the exercise physiologist who will conduct the test. Kaitlyn reviews LeRoy's chart and determines his pre-test likelihood of ischemic heart disease. She refers to the chart, and as Le Roy is a man 60 to 69 years of age with typical angina she determines he has a high likelihood of ischemic heart disease. This is useful information to know before conducting the graded exercise test.

After conducting the test, Kaitlyn begins to write the report. She notes LeRoy reached a workload of 10 METs, at which he stopped because of chest pain (3 on the 4-point scale). Reviewing the electrocardiogram (ECG), Kaitlyn finds LeRoy has 2 mm of ST-segment depression. Using this information and the Duke Nomogram, she draws a straight line from 2 mm ST-segment deviation to exercise-limiting angina during exercise. She finds where this line intersects the ischemic-reading line. Kaitlyn then draws a straight line from this intersection to 10 on the exercise METs scale. She then reads the prognosis, which is about a 4% annual mortality and a five-year survival rate of 0.80, or 80%.

Demonstration Case Study 4.2

Clinical exercise testing and interpretation

Beth is the director of exercise testing at a local hospital. Knowing that exercise testing is not perfect because there are sometimes false negatives and false positives, Beth collects data on 100 patients who have been tested recently. She looks at the graded exercise tests and the follow-up diagnostic tests that have been done. She finds the following:

47 True positives

44 True negatives

3 False positives

6 False negatives

She first computes the sensitivity or percentage of those who test positive and have ischemic heart disease:

$$\text{Sensitivity} = [TP/(TP + FN)] \times 100\%$$
$$= [47/(47 + 6)] \times 100\%$$
$$= [47/53] \times 100\%$$
$$= 0.887 \times 100\%$$
$$= 88.7\%$$

To find the specificity or the percentage of those who test negative and do not have ischemic heart disease Beth does the following:

$$\text{Specificity} = [TN/(FP + TN)] \times 100\%$$
$$= [44/(3 + 44)] \times 100\%$$
$$= [44/47] \times 100\%$$
$$= 0.936 \times 100\%$$
$$= 93.6\%$$

Next, she calculates the positive predictive value or the percentage of positive tests that were true positives:

$$\text{Positive predictive value} = [TP/(TP + FP)] \times 100\%$$
$$= [47/(47 + 3)] \times 100\%$$
$$= [47/50] \times 100\%$$
$$= 0.940 \times 100\%$$
$$= 94.0\%$$

Last, Beth determines the negative predictive value or the percentage of negative tests that were true negatives:

$$\text{Negative predictive value} = [TN/(TN + FN)] \times 100\%$$
$$= [44/44 + 6] \times 100\%$$
$$= [44/50] \times 100\%$$
$$= 0.880 \times 100\%$$
$$= 88.0\%$$

Student Case Study 4.1

Clinical exercise testing and interpretation

Matilda is a 59-year-old woman who is referred for a graded exercise test. She has been experiencing episodes of dizziness and her physician wants to see if it may be heart related. She has not had any chest pain (angina). During the test she is able to attain 13 METs. She has no chest pain or ST-segment deviation.

1. Determine her pre-test likelihood of ischemic heart disease.
2. Determine her post-test prognosis.

Student Case Study 4.2

Clinical exercise testing and interpretation

Gregory is a 49-year-old man who has episodic pain in the chest that is believed to be gastrointestinal and not angina. Because of his poor fitness level he has been referred to a clinic for a graded exercise test. In the test he achieves 5 METs, at which point he is very short of breath and cannot continue the test. His ECG reveals he has 2 mm of ST-segment depression and he had slight chest pain that does not cause him to stop the test.

1. Determine his pre-test likelihood of ischemic heart disease.
2. Determine his post-test prognosis.

Student Case Study 4.3

Clinical exercise testing and interpretation

A clinic that does graded exercise testing wants to know the effectiveness of the testing or the diagnostic value. After reviewing 100 cases they find the following:

40 True positives

42 True negatives

7 False positives

11 False negatives

1. Determine the sensitivity of the testing at the facility.
2. Determine the specificity of the testing at the facility.
3. Determine the positive predictive value of the testing at the facility.
4. Determine the negative predictive value of the testing at the facility.

Student Case Study 4.4

Clinical exercise testing and interpretation

A second clinic that does graded exercise testing wants to know the effectiveness of the testing or the diagnostic value. After reviewing 100 cases they find the following:

39 True positives

40 True negatives

11 False positives

10 False negatives

1. Determine the sensitivity of the testing at the facility.
2. Determine the specificity of the testing at the facility.
3. Determine the positive predictive value of the testing at the facility.
4. Determine the negative predictive value of the testing at the facility.

REFERENCES

1. Gibbons RJ, Balady GJ, Bricker JT, et al. ACC/AHA 2002 guideline update for exercise testing: summary article. A report of the American College of Cardiology/American Heart Association Task Force on Practice Guidelines (Committee to Update the 1997 Exercise teasing Guidelines). *J Am Coll Cardiol* 40(8): 1531–1540, 2002.

2. Mark DB, Shaw L, Harrell FE Jr, et al. Prognostic value of a treadmill exercise score in outpatients with expected coronary artery disease. *N Engl J Med* 325(12): 849–853, 1991.

CHAPTER 5

Metabolic Equations

INTRODUCTION

MANY PEOPLE USE cardio exercise equipment such as treadmills, stationary bicycles, and stepping machines to improve their fitness levels. With computerization, these types of equipment are capable of displaying data about the workout that includes exercise time, speed, distance, heart rate and kilocalories burned. While some of these values are easy to determine, some require calculations developed from research. In this chapter the calculations for determining oxygen consumption ($\dot{V}O_2$), metabolic equivalents (METs), and kilocalories burned will be considered.

To work through the case studies and problems presented students will need to understand the equations for calculating oxygen consumption for walking, running, stepping, leg cycling, and arm cycling. The equations for each of these activities have three components: resting, horizontal, and vertical. Some problems will require the calculation of oxygen consumption or kilocalories and some will require the calculation of the settings for speed, grade, or resistance to obtain a target $\dot{V}O_2$.

The purpose of this chapter is to teach students how to use the metabolic equations to compute energy expenditures. On completion of the case studies, students will be able to:

1. Calculate oxygen consumption for different workloads on common exercise equipment
2. Determine specific workload settings to match exercise prescription workload intensities
3. Estimate caloric expenditures for various workloads
4. Compute metabolic equivalents (METs) for common exercise activities

WALKING ON A TREADMILL

The variables that determine the oxygen consumption while walking are the speed and the grade of the treadmill. For the metabolic equations the unit of measure for the speed of the treadmill is meters per minute. Because most treadmills display miles per hour, the speed must be converted by multiplying miles per hour by 26.8 to get meters per minute.

To calculate the $\dot{V}O_2$ of walking on a treadmill the resting, horizontal, and vertical components of the activity must be summed[1]:

$$VO_2 \text{ (mL/kg-min)} = [3.5 + (0.1 \times speed) + (1.8 \times speed \times grade)]$$

The resting component is the oxygen consumption at rest, which is equal to 3.5 mL/kg-min or 1 MET. To get the horizontal component, the speed of the treadmill in meters per minute is multiplied by 0.1. The vertical component is equal to the speed in meters per minute times 1.8 times the grade of the treadmill. The grade of the treadmill is a percent and the percent must be converted to decimal form (5% grade equals 0.05). Examples of these calculations are found in the case studies.

RUNNING ON A TREADMILL

The running formula is similar in structure to the walking formula. The speed and grade are measured in the same way. The resting component is the same. The equation is the sum of the resting, horizontal, and vertical components[2]:

$$VO_2 \text{ (mL/kg-min)} = [3.5 + (0.2 \times speed) + (0.9 \times speed \times grade)]$$

The difference between the running and walking formulas is that the coefficient for the horizontal component is 0.2 for running and 0.1 for walking, and the coefficient of the vertical component is 0.9 for running and 1.8 for walking.

Walking is defined as having at least one foot on the ground at all times while running is not having both feet on the ground at any time. For the purposes of these formulas walking is most accurate between 1.9 and 3.7 miles per hour. Running is most accurate at more than 5 miles per hour. This leaves a gap between 3.7 and 5 miles per hour. Generally if the person is jogging at these speeds the running formula would be used.

STEPPING

The formula for stepping involves going up and a down a single step. The variables that determine work rate are the height of the step and the stepping rate. The step height is measured in meters and the rate in steps per minute. One step is four counts, right leg up, left leg up, right leg down, left leg down. When using a metronome to control the stepping rate the metronome should be set at four times the stepping rate.

The formula for stepping includes the same three components: walking, running, and resting, horizontal and vertical:[3]

$$VO_2 \text{ (mL/kg-min)} = [3.5 + (0.2 \times steps/min) + (1.33 \times (1.8 \times step\ height \times steps/min))]$$

The 1.33 accounts for going up and down. Going down with gravity requires one third of the energy (0.33) of going up against gravity (1.0).

CYCLING ON A LEG ERGOMETER

There are two major differences between cycling and walking, running or stepping. The first is sitting versus standing during the exercise. When sitting during cycling the exercisers do not support their own body weight. Because people have different body weights the absolute energy expenditure is more for heavier people when supporting their own weight in a standing position such as walking, running and stepping. During cycling the energy expenditure is the same for people of any weight when the workload is the same. The second difference is that gravity is not a factor in the work rate. The work rate is determined by the resistance on the flywheel over time. Therefore, there is no vertical component and instead there is a resistance component. There is still a resting component of 3.5 mL/kg-min and a horizontal component of 3.5. The formula for leg cycling is[4]:

$$VO_2 \text{ (mL/kg-min)} = [3.5 + 3.5 + ((1.8 \times \text{work rate})/\text{body weight})]$$

The work rate is determined by the resistance on the flywheel times the pedal rate in revolutions per minute times the distance through which the resistance is applied. The resistance is set on the ergometer and measured in kilograms. The pedal rate is measured in revolutions per minute. The type of ergometer determines the size of the flywheel. Monark ergometers have a 6-meter flywheel while Tunturi and BodyGuard ergometers have a 3-meter flywheel. The work rate is measured in kilogram meters per minute (kg-m/min).

Because riders do not support their own body weight the work rate is divided by their body weight in kilograms. Therefore, the formula can be reduced to[5]:

$$VO_2 \text{ (mL/kg-min)} = [7.0 + ((1.8 \times \text{work rate})/\text{body weight})]$$

CYCLING ON AN ARM ERGOMETER

For individuals who have limitations in the lower body such as back or knee injuries, an arm ergometer can be used. The arm cycle ergometer formula is similar to that for the leg cycle ergometer. The main difference is that there is no horizontal component. The equation is[6]:

$$VO_2 \text{ (mL/kg-min)} = [3.5 + ((3 \times \text{work rate})/\text{body weight})]$$

The formula for the work rate is the same as for the leg ergometer: resistance times revolutions per minute times the flywheel distance. The main arm ergometer used is the Monark, which has a flywheel of 2.4 meters. Since the arms have less muscle mass than the legs, the work rate is lower in arm ergometers than in leg ergometers. The kilograms of resistance and the flywheel size are less.

METABOLIC EQUIVALENTS

Oxygen consumption is measured in milliliters of oxygen consumed per kilogram of body weight per minute (ml/kg-min), liters of oxygen consumed per minute (L/min), or metabolic equivalent (METs). One MET equals 3.5 mL/kg-min of oxygen consumption for the average person at rest. All people are different and some may have slightly higher or lower values. However, when converting a $\dot{V}O_2$ to METs the $\dot{V}O_2$ in mL/kg-min is divided by 3.5. METs gives a number that indicates how many times the oxygen consumption is compared to that at rest.

CALORIC EXPENDITURE

When the oxygen consumption is known the caloric expenditure can be calculated. Because oxygen is used to burn fats and carbohydrates aerobically there is a correlation between amount of oxygen burned and the amount of kilocalories burned. (Calories is the term used in lay communication but it is actually kilocalories.) The actual amount of kilocalories burned depends on how much is from fat and how much is from carbohydrates. However, for simplicity the conversion generally used is that 1 liter of oxygen consumed is equal to 4.9 kilocalories burned. When calculating caloric consumption during exercise, the weight of the individual and the amount of time spent exercising must be considered. Those with a higher body weight will burn more energy and the longer one exercises the more energy that is burned.

Demonstration Case Study 5.1

Metabolic equations

Cihan is a 170-pound man who typically rides a Monark leg ergometer at 70 rpm with 3 kg of resistance for 30 minutes as part of his regular workout. For his convenience, he exercises at home in his basement. He decided to join a fitness club that opened near his house because he wants to try using a treadmill. During his orientation with his trainer Alicia, he asks what would be an equivalent workload on a treadmill to his current cycling workload. Alicia said she could figure that out.

First Alicia has to determine his oxygen consumption on the Monark. She converts his weight to kilograms by dividing his weight in pounds by 2.2 (170/2.2 = 77.3 kg). She then determines the work rate of the Monark, which has a 6-meter flywheel.

Work rate = resistance (kg) × revolutions per minute × flywheel meters per revolution

= 3 kg × 70 rpm × 6 m/rev

= 1260 kg-m/min

Using the work rate she then calculates the oxygen consumption using the leg cycling formula.

$$VO_2 = 7 + (1.8 \times \text{work rate})/\text{body weight}$$
$$= 7 + [(1.8 \times 1260)/77.3]$$
$$= 7 + (2268/77.3)$$
$$= 7 + 29.3$$
$$= 36.3 \text{ mL/kg-min}$$

Now Alicia calculates the speed of the treadmill, which equals 36.3 mL/kg-min using the running formula.

$$VO_2 = 3.5 + 0.2 \times \text{speed of the treadmill}$$
$$36.3 \text{ mL/kg-min} = 3.5 + 0.2 \times \text{speed}$$
$$32.8 = 0.2 \times \text{speed}$$
$$164 \text{ m/min} = \text{speed}$$

Cihan asks what the speed is in miles per hour. Alicia converts meters per minute to miles per hour by dividing by 26.8.

$$164/26.8 = 6.1 \text{ miles per hour}$$

Cihan goes over to the treadmill and sets it at 6.1 miles per hour. He starts running and is not comfortable. He goes back to Alicia and says he thinks he would rather walk. Alicia says this is possible but to reach that workload he would need to add some grade. He could not walk on flat ground and reach the $\dot{V}O_2$ equivalent to that of the cycling. Alicia recalculates using the walking formula at a 10% grade.

$$VO_2 = 3.5 + 0.1 \times \text{speed} + 1.8 \times \text{speed} \times \text{grade}$$
$$36.3 \text{ mL/kg-min} = 3.5 + (0.1 \times \text{speed}) + (1.8 \times \text{speed} \times 0.1)$$
$$36.3 = 3.5 + (0.1 \times \text{speed}) + (0.18 \times \text{speed})$$
$$32.8 = (0.1 \times \text{speed}) + (0.18 \times \text{speed})$$
$$32.8 = 0.28 \times \text{speed}$$
$$117.1 \text{ m/min} = \text{speed}$$

Alicia converts this to miles per hour.

$$117.1/26.8 = 4.4 \text{ miles per hour}$$

She tells Cihan that at 10% grade this is a very fast walk. If he really wants to walk the grade will need to be increased. She then calculates a new speed using 12% grade.

$$VO_2 = 3.5 + 0.1 \times \text{speed} + 1.8 \times \text{speed} \times \text{grade}$$
$$36.3 \text{ mL/kg-min} = 3.5 + (0.1 \times \text{speed}) + (1.8 \times \text{speed} \times 0.12)$$

36.3 = 3.5 + (0.1 × speed) + (0.22 × speed)

32.8 = (0.1 × speed) + (0.22 × speed)

32.8 = 0.32 × speed

102.5 m/min = speed

Alicia converts this to miles per hour.

102.5/26.8 = 3.8 miles per hour

Cihan tries walking on the treadmill at 3.8 miles per hour at 12% grade and decided this was more comfortable and a speed he could stick with. Then he asked how many kilocalories he would burn in a workout if he walked at this pace and grade for 40 minutes. Alicia calculated this by first converting his weight to kilograms.

170 pounds/2.2 = 77.3 kilograms

36.3 mL/kg-min × 1 L/1000 mL × 77.3 kg × 40 min × 4.9 kcal/L = 550.0 kilocalories

Cihan thinks this is great. If he works out four times per week he can burn 2,000 kilocalories! That would really help his weight-loss goals.

Student Case Study 5.1

Metabolic equations

Julianna does a step test to exhaustion on a 25-cm step and stops because of leg fatigue at a stepping rate of 30 steps per minute. She would like to know her estimated $\dot{V}O_{2max}$ based on the test. She would also like to know her maximum METs.

1. Calculate her volume of oxygen consumed at maximum exercise.
2. Convert her $\dot{V}O_{2max}$ to maxMETs.

Student Case Study 5.2

Metabolic equations

Jon weighs 70 kg and wants to know if he would burn more kilocalories walking 3.5 miles per hour at 5% grade for 30 minutes, five times per week or running 6 miles per hour at 5% grade for 30 minutes, three times per week.

1. Calculate his weekly kilocalories burned walking 3.5 miles per hour at 5% grade for 30 minutes, five times per week.
2. Calculate his weekly kilocalories burned running 6 miles per hour at 5% grade for 30 minutes, three times per week.
3. Indicate which activity will burn more kilocalories per week.

Student Case Study 5.3

Liang weighs 155 pounds and wants to ride his BodyGuard cycle ergometer at 10 METs. He would like to know the revolutions per minute and resistance he should use. He would like to vary his workout by changing the resistance among 5, 6, 7, and 8 kg. He wants to know the corresponding revolutions per minute.

1. Calculate the revolutions per minute with 5 kg resistance to equal 10 METs on a BodyGuard cycle ergometer.
2. Calculate the revolutions per minute with 6 kg resistance to equal 10 METs on a BodyGuard cycle ergometer.
3. Calculate the revolutions per minute with 7 kg resistance to equal 10 METs on a BodyGuard cycle ergometer.
4. Calculate the revolutions per minute with 8 kg resistance to equal 10 METs on a BodyGuard cycle ergometer.

Student Case Study 5.4

Peter weighs 160 pounds and is a long-time runner who recently had knee-replacement surgery. His general health is excellent and he wants to maintain it by continuing some form of exercise. At his rehab clinic he learned about the Monark arm ergometer. Before his surgery, he was riding a Monark leg ergometer at 60 revolutions per minute and 3.5 kg of resistance. He wants to know the equivalent resistance on the arm ergometer at 70 revolutions per minute.

1. Calculate the $\dot{V}O_2$ for riding a Monark leg ergometer at 60 revolutions per minute and 3.5 kg of resistance.
2. Calculate the resistance needed on the arm ergometer at 70 revolutions per minute to equal the $\dot{V}O_2$ for riding a Monark leg ergometer at 60 revolutions per minute and 3.5 kg of resistance.

Student Case Study 5.5

Jenna weighs 192 pounds and likes to walk at the local mall, which has a flat walking surface. She prefers to walk at a speed of 3 miles per hour. She heard that to lose weight she should burn 2,000 kilocalories per week doing aerobic exercise. She wants to know how many minutes she needs to exercise each week to meet this goal.

(Because the walking surface is flat the treadmill equation can be used to estimate her calories burned.)

1. Calculate her $\dot{V}O_2$ for walking 3 miles per hour at 0% grade.
2. Calculate how many minutes she needs to exercise per week to burn 2,000 kilocalories.

REFERENCES

1. American College of Sports Medicine. *ACSM's Guidelines for Exercise Testing and Prescription,* 11th edition. Philadelphia, PA: Wolters Kluwer Health, 2022.
2. ibid.
3. ibid.
4. ibid.
5. ibid.
6. ibid.

CHAPTER 6

FITT-VP Principle for Cardiorespiratory Endurance

INTRODUCTION

AN EXERCISE PROGRAM aimed at improving overall health should include cardiorespiratory endurance training. This type of exercise is continuous and rhythmical, using the major muscle groups. When done properly it stresses the cardiovascular and respiratory systems to improve the delivery of oxygen to the working muscles.

Before attempting to write exercise prescriptions for cardiorespiratory endurance, students should review the FITT-VP principles and guidelines. (FITT is an acronym for Frequency, Intensity, Time, and Type of exercise; VP is an acronym for Volume and Progression.) Special attention should be given to the formulas for determining exercise intensity (see Chapter 5). However, all components of the FITT-VP must be understood before writing the exercise prescriptions in the case studies presented.

The purpose of this chapter is to teach students how to design the cardiorespiratory endurance portion of an exercise program. On completion of the case studies, students will be able to:

1. Determine the appropriate number of days per week to exercise
2. Calculate the exercise intensity using the following methods:
    a. Heart rate reserve
    b. Oxygen consumption ($\dot{V}O_2$) reserve
    c. Heart rate
    d. $\dot{V}O_2$
    e. Metabolic equivalents (METs)
3. Establish the exercise time per session
4. Recommend the effective mode of exercise
5. Incorporate the correct volume of physical activity
6. Adapt the exercise program for continuous progress
7. Explain the components of the exercise session.

COMPONENTS OF THE EXERCISE SESSION

Whatever the type of training program being performed, each exercise session should include four basic phases: warm-up, conditioning, cool-down, and stretching. The conditioning component is the major one and the exercise prescriptions discussed later will address the specific design.

Warm-up. Before stressing the heart, lungs, and muscles during the conditioning phase of a workout, exercisers must progressively prepare the body. Less than 15 minutes of lower intensity exercise such as walking or jogging will slowly increase the body temperature, heart rate, and breathing, which will help the body transition to the conditioning phase. In general, when exercisers break a light sweat the body is warmed up and ready for more intense activities.

Cool-down. After the conditioning phase of the exercise session has been completed it is important to gradually move the body toward rest. Maintaining the muscle pump with lower level activities such as walking for 5 to 10 minutes will allow the heart rate and blood pressure to decrease slowly while continuing to remove lactic acid and other byproducts accumulated during the workout. This may aid recovery.

Stretching. The best time to stretch is when the body is warm, making the end of a workout a good time. Stretching can be part of the warm-up but most believe the end of the cool-down is the best time to improve flexibility. At least 10 minutes of stretching is recommended. The specific recommendations for developing flexibility will be presented in Chapter 8.

CARDIORESPIRATORY ENDURANCE CONDITIONING

When writing an exercise prescription for the conditioning phase of a cardiorespiratory (or aerobic) workout program the FITT-VP principles should be used.[1] Most of the attention is given to intensity. However, frequency, type of exercise, and time are also important. The volume of exercise and progression must also be considered.

Intensity. The intensity of the workload can be monitored in different ways. The easiest for most exercisers to understand is heart rate. Two formulas are used for heart rate prescriptions: the heart rate reserve and heart rate methods. The heart rate reserve method uses maximum or peak heart rate and resting heart rate while the heart rate method uses maximum or peak heart rate only. The desired percent intensity for each method must be decided. The guidelines are clearer for the heart rate reserve method, where moderate exercise is defined as 40% to 59% and vigorous is greater than 60%. If light exercise is desired then 30% to 39% would be used. There is some flexibility in selecting the specific percent ranges but it is important to stay within the broad, general guidelines.

Intensity prescriptions can also be written using maximum volume of oxygen consumed or the oxygen consumed reserve, which is the maximum volume of oxygen consumed minus the resting oxygen consumption (3.5 mL/kg-min). The recommended percentages for the oxygen consumption reserve method are the same as for the heart rate reserve method.

When neither the heart rate nor oxygen consumption methods are logical, the 6–20 Rating of Perceived Exertion (RPE) Scale can be used.[2] Using the RPE Scale 9–11 is light intensity, 12–13 is moderate intensity, and greater than 14 is vigorous intensity. One example of when the RPE Scale is better to use during later months of pregnancy.

Frequency. How often exercisers should do cardiorespiratory training workouts per week depends on the intensity and time of the workout. Moderate-intensity exercise should be done at least five days per week and vigorous-intensity exercise should be done at least three days per week. Equivalent combinations of the two, such as two days each of moderate- and vigorous-intensity exercise, are also acceptable. These can be further modified based on the time of the exercise sessions. See "Volume" below for more specific combinations.

Time and pattern. The duration of the conditioning phase of a single aerobic workout day should be 30 to 60 minutes of moderate-intensity exercise or 20 to 60 minutes of vigorous-intensity exercise. Ideally the pattern would be continuous but the total time may be broken into short intervals of 10 to 15 minutes if exercisers are unable to go the full time at once. In general, any length of exercise time is better than none. The goal should be to gradually increase the interval times until the full recommendation can be met.

Type. The mode of exercise chosen for the workout should include activities that the exercisers enjoy. The American College of Sports Medicine distributes exercise types into four different groups[3]. Group A activities are appropriate for all adults and include walking and slow cycling. Group B activities require little skill but more physical fitness to perform. This includes higher-intensity activities such as jogging, running, and fast cycling. Group C activities require skill such as swimming and skating. Group D activities include recreational sports such as soccer, basketball, and tennis. The general recommendations for exercise type are: beginners should start with Group A and progress as fitness and skills are developed; adults with at least average fitness can do Group B and C activities for which they have skills; and adults who have at least average fitness and maintain a regular exercise program can participate in Group D activities.

Volume. The total amount of aerobic exercise recommended per week can be measured several ways as a measure of energy expenditure. One is the MET-min, which is the minutes of exercise times the MET level of that exercise. When computed for one week there may be several different types of exercise at different MET (intensity) levels that need to be summed together. The recommendation is more than 500 to 1000 MET-min per week.

Another measure of volume is kilocalories burned per week. To obtain health benefits a minimum of 1,000 kilocalories from moderate physical activity should be burned each week. Some people like to use step counters. Although the accuracy of these instruments can vary greatly, it is recommended that exercisers step at least 7,000 to 8,000 times per day. A simpler method is to log about 150 minutes per week of moderate-intensity activity. Given that exercise volume is altered by changing either exercise frequency, intensity, or time, exercise prescriptions that have the correct frequency, intensity, and time will also be the correct volume.

Progression. Once an exercise prescription is written the work is not done. As exercisers' bodies adapt to the stress of exercise their exercise prescription must be modified. Considering the overload principle of training the exercise prescription needs to be changed in order to obtain more benefits. The important consideration is to progress slowly. The heart-rate prescription methods for intensity work well because they do not have to change. As the exercisers become more fit, they can work out at higher levels without seeing an increase in the workout heart rate due to physiological adaptations. However, they may need to increase the frequency or time of exercise to continue to make the desired improvements and obtain additional health benefits.

Demonstration Case Study 6.1

Cardiorespiratory endurance

Maddie is a 40-year-old, healthy woman who wants to start an endurance-training program. She meets with Jim, an exercise physiologist, and he conducts a graded exercise treadmill test using the Bruce protocol. Maddie's resting values are: heart rate 73 beats per minute (bpm) and blood pressure 128/70 mm Hg. Her weight is 151 pounds. She completes the third stage of the test, which is 3.4 miles per hour at 14% grade. The max values on the treadmill were: heart rate 182 bpm, blood pressure 180/72 mm Hg, RPE 20, and an estimated 10.1 METs. Jim starts by considering the intensity of exercise. Maddie indicated that her goal is to run for at least 45 minutes. Because she is basically sedentary, Jim decides to start her walking at a moderate intensity of 50% to 60% of heart rate reserve. He calculates her heart rate prescription:

Heart Rate Reserve (HRR) = Max Heart Rate (MHR) – Resting Heart Rate (RHR)

HRR = 182 – 73

HRR = 109 bpm

Minimum HRR prescription = HRR × 0.5 + RHR

Maximum HRR prescription = HRR × 0.6 + RHR

Minimum HRR prescription = 109 × 0.5 + 73 = 128 bpm

Maximum HRR prescription = 109 × 0.6 + 73 = 138 bpm

Because Jim has prescribed a moderate intensity of exercise he decides to increase her frequency from the minimum of three days per week to five. He chooses to start her exercise time at 30 minutes per workout. Then she will meet the weekly recommendation of 150 minutes per week of moderate-intensity exercise.

After writing the prescription Jim meets with Maddie to describe her program. Because her goal is to run and she has not exercised regularly in the past he recommends starting with a Group A activity such as walking. She can progress to a Group B activity such as jogging when she develops a greater aerobic base. He explains that she should wear her heart rate monitor while walking and check it periodically to confirm she is at a walking pace where her heart rate stays between 128 and 138 bpm. He further explains that if her heart rate drops below 128 bpm she needs to walk faster and if it rises above 138 bpm she needs to walk slower. This pace will provide a good training effect and improve her health. Jim also tells her that she needs to walk at that pace for 30 minutes each time she works out and she needs to work out five times per week. Jim further explains that she should always begin with a 5- to 10-minute warm-up to prepare her body for the workout. This should include slow walking before her faster workout pace. After the conditioning portion she should do a cool-down of 5 to 10 minutes of slower walking and then 10 minutes of stretching. They talk about a schedule of days and times that will work for her.

Maddie is concerned that she really wants to run and she is being advised to walk. Jim clarifies that her body will adapt to the exercise better if she starts slow and gradually progresses to higher intensities. Maddie thinks about the exercise prescription. She says the weather is a little cold and she would prefer to start inside on a treadmill. She also likes the idea of watching television while working out and does not want to keep checking her pulse. She asks Jim for another way to monitor her exercise intensity. Jim calculates a new intensity prescription based on $\dot{V}O_2$ by first converting her maxMETs to $\dot{V}O_{2max}$.

Resting VO_2 = 3.5 mL/kg-min (1 MET at rest)

VO_{2max} = 10.1 METs × 3.5 mL/kg-min

VO_{2max} = 35.4 mL/kg-min

Then Jim calculates the intensity prescription using the $\dot{V}O_2$ Reserve Method.

VO_2 Reserve = VO_{2max} – VO_{2Rest}

VO_2 Reserve = 35.4 mL/kg-min – 3.5 mL/kg-min

VO_2 Reserve = 31.9 mL/kg-min

Jim then uses the same percentages as the heart rate prescription to calculate the moderate intensity of exercise.

Minimum VO_2 prescription = VO_2 Reserve × 0.5 + 3.5

Maximum VO_2 prescription = VO_2 Reserve × 0.6 + 3.5

Minimum VO_2 prescription = 31.9 × 0.5 + 3.5 = 19.5 mL/kg-min

Maximum VO_2 prescription = 31.9 × 0.6 + 3.5 = 22.6 mL/kg-min

Now that Jim has the $\dot{V}O_2$ prescription he has to do some calculations to make it understandable for Maddie. He refers back to the metabolic equations. Using the walking formula he calculates the speed of the treadmill using a 0% grade.

VO_2 = 3.5 + 0.1 × speed + 1.8 × speed × grade

19.5 mL/kg-min = 3.5 + (0.1 × speed) + (1.8 × speed × 0)

19.5 = 3.5 + (0.1 × speed)

16.0 = (0.1 × speed)

160.0 m/min = speed

Jim converts this to miles per hour.

160.0/26.8 = 6.0 miles per hour

Therefore, the minimum speed would be 6.0 miles per hour. Then Jim calculates the maximum speed.

$VO_2 = 3.5 + 0.1 \times speed + 1.8 \times speed \times grade$

$22.6 \text{ mL/kg-min} = 3.5 + (0.1 \times speed) + (1.8 \times speed \times 0)$

$22.6 = 3.5 + (0.1 \times speed)$

$19.1 = (0.1 \times speed)$

$191.0 \text{ m/min} = speed$

Jim converts this to miles per hour.

$191.0/26.8 = 7.1 \text{ miles per hour}$

Now his recommendation to Maddie is to walk on the treadmill between 6.0 and 7.1 miles per hour. However, Jim knows that 6.0 miles per hour is clearly a running speed. He must increase the grade from 0% in order to obtain a walking speed. Jim decides to try a 5% grade.

$VO_2 = 3.5 + 0.1 \times speed + 1.8 \times speed \times grade$

$19.5 \text{ mL/kg-min} = 3.5 + (0.1 \times speed) + (1.8 \times speed \times 0.05)$

$19.5 = 3.5 + (0.1 \times speed) + (1.8 \times speed \times 0.05)$

$16.0 = (0.1 \times speed) + (0.09 \times speed)$

$16.0 = (0.19 \times speed)$

$84.2 \text{ m/min} = speed$

Jim converts this to miles per hour.

$84.2/26.8 = 3.1 \text{ miles per hour}$

The new minimum walking speed is 3.1 miles per hour and this is a true walking speed. The new maximum walking speed is calculated next.

$VO_2 = 3.5 + 0.1 \times speed + 1.8 \times speed \times grade$

$22.6 \text{ mL/kg-min} = 3.5 + (0.1 \times speed) + (1.8 \times speed \times 0.05)$

$22.6 = 3.5 + (0.1 \times speed) + (1.8 \times speed \times 0.05)$

$19.1 = (0.1 \times speed) + (0.09 \times speed)$

$19.1 = (0.19 \times speed)$

$100.5 \text{ m/min} = speed$

Jim converts this to miles per hour.

$100.5/26.8 = 3.8 \text{ miles per hour}$

Based on these computations Jim tells Maddie that she should walk on the treadmill between 3.1 and 3.8 miles per hour at 5% grade. He recommends 3.5 miles per hour as a starting point. Maddie thinks that sounds good. She asks how many calories she would burn each week. (Most people say calories but Jim knows she actually is interested in kilocalories.) Jim starts by converting her weight to kilograms.

151 pounds/2.2 = 68.6 kilograms

Jim next converts the speed in miles per hour to meters per minute.

3.5 miles per hour × 26.8 = 93.8 meters per minute

Then he computes the $\dot{V}O_2$.

VO_2 = 3.5 + 0.1 × speed + 1.8 × speed × grade
VO_2 = 3.5 + (0.1 × 93.8) + (1.8 × 93.8 × 0.05)
VO_2 = 3.5 + (9.38) + (8.44)
VO_2 = 21.3 mL/kg-min

Because there are about 4.9 kilocalories per liter of oxygen consumed Jim does the following assuming she walks at 3.5 miles per hour at 5% grade for 30 minutes at each workout.

21.3 mL/kg-min × 1 L/1,000 mL × 68.6 kg × 30 min × 4.9 kcal/L = 214.8 kilocalories

Doing this workout five times per week will result in 1,096 kilocalories burned per week.

214.8 kcal/workout × 5 workouts/week = 1.074.0 kcal/week

Since Jim has these numbers he decides to verify the volume of work in MET-min/week. He starts with the $\dot{V}O_2$ prescribed (21.3 mL/kg-min).

21.3 mL/kg-min/3.5 mL/kg-min = 6.1 METs

5 workouts/week × 30 min/workout = 150 min/week

6.1 METs × 150 min/week = 915 MET-min/week. This is sufficient to meet the volume guideline of 500 – 1,000 MET-min/week.

Maddie is happy with her prescription and looks forward to progressing from walking to running. Jim concludes by explaining that this prescription is the conditioning portion of her program. She should always start with a 5-to 10-minute warm-up such as a slow walk and gradually stretch her muscles by progressively increasing her strides to a comfortable length. She should also feel her body temperature rising and notice sweat beginning to form on her forehead. Then she is ready to begin her conditioning.

After Maddie completes the 30-minute conditioning program she should do a 5- to 10-minute cool-down. Jim recommends slowing down the walking pace during this time to allow the heart rate to gradually decline and keep her leg muscles contracting to help the blood return to the heart against gravity. This should be followed by 10 minutes of stretching to improve flexibility. That concludes a typical exercise training session.

Cardiorespiratory endurance

Katrina is 24 years old. She goes to the YMCA fitness center and is given a cardiorespiratory endurance exercise prescription. For the conditioning part of her program she is instructed to use cardio machines of her choice for 30 minutes, four times per week, and maintain a heart rate between 137 and 167 bpm. Explain the other components that make up the exercise training session besides conditioning.

1. Describe activities should she do before the conditioning component and why.
2. Describe activities should she do immediately after the conditioning component and why.
3. Describe activities she should do for flexibility.

Student Case Study 6.2

Cardiorespiratory endurance

Jorge is a 36-year-old, healthy man who wants to step up his running program. He meets with an exercise physiologist who conducts a screening and graded exercise treadmill test using the Bruce protocol. Jorge is cleared for vigorous exercise. Jorge's resting values are: heart rate 66 bpm and blood pressure 118/68 mm Hg. His weight is 191 pounds. He completes the fourth stage of the test, which is 4.2 miles per hour at 16% grade. The max values on the treadmill were: heart rate 185 bpm, blood pressure 188/68 mm Hg, RPE 19, and an estimated 12.9 METs. Determine the exercise prescription by considering the FITT-VP principle.

1. Calculate a heart rate prescription for vigorous exercise using the heart rate reserve method.
2. Calculate a prescription for vigorous exercise using the $\dot{V}O_2$ reserve method.
3. Indicate which aerobic exercise group should be used for the type of exercise that should be performed.
4. Determine the frequency of cardiorespiratory training.
5. Recommend the time of training for the exercise session.
6. Verify whether the prescription is the appropriate volume.
7. Comment on the pattern of the training.
8. Discuss progression for continued overload and improvement.
9. Explain the make-up of the entire exercise session which includes before and after the conditioning phase.

Jane is a 26-year-old woman who wants to start a cardiorespiratory endurance training program. During four years of playing college soccer she suffered multiple knee injuries. She is no longer able to run and has a difficult time walking short distances. She meets with an exercise physiologist who conducts a screening and graded exercise test using a leg ergometer that she tolerated well. Jane is cleared for vigorous exercise. Jane's resting values are: heart rate 71 bpm and blood pressure 106/58 mm Hg. Her weight is 143 pounds. She completes the submax YMCA bicycle test. Using her estimated maximum heart rate, the data from her test were projected to a maximum work rate of 1,150 kpm/min. Determine the exercise prescription by considering the FITT-VP principle.

1. Calculate a heart rate prescription for vigorous exercise using the heart rate reserve method.
2. Calculate a prescription for vigorous exercise using the $\dot{V}O_2$ reserve method.
3. Indicate which aerobic exercise group should be used for the type of exercise that should be performed.
4. Determine the frequency of cardiorespiratory training.
5. Recommend the time of training for the exercise session.
6. Verify whether the prescription is the appropriate volume.
7. Comment on the pattern of the training.
8. Discuss progression for continued overload and improvement.
9. Explain the make-up of the entire exercise session which includes before and after the conditioning phase.

Student Case Study 6.4

Richard is an 18-year-old, healthy man who wants to get more information about his cardiorespiratory exercise program. He meets with an exercise physiologist at the campus recreation center. Richard is cleared for vigorous exercise. His resting values are: heart rate 60 bpm and blood pressure 116/70 mm Hg. His weight is 169 pounds. Richard completes the 12-minute walk/run test. His $\dot{V}O_{2max}$ was estimated to be 48 mL/kg-min. Determine the exercise prescription by considering the FITT-VP principle.

1. Calculate a heart rate prescription for vigorous exercise using the heart rate reserve method.
2. Calculate a prescription for vigorous exercise using the $\dot{V}O_2$ reserve method.
3. Indicate which aerobic exercise group should be used for the type of exercise that should be performed.

4. Determine the frequency of cardiorespiratory training.
5. Recommend the time of training for the exercise session.
6. Verify whether the prescription is the appropriate volume.
7. Comment on the pattern of the training.
8. Discuss progression for continued overload and improvement.
9. Explain the make-up of the entire exercise session which includes before and after the conditioning phase.

REFERENCES

1. Borg, GA. Perceived exertion. *Exerc Sport Sci Rev.* 2: 131–153, 1974.

2. ibid.

3. American College of Sports Medicine. *ACSM's Guidelines for Exercise Testing and Prescription*, 11th edition. Philadelphia, PA: Wolters Kluwer Health, 2022.

CHAPTER 7

FITT-VP Principle for Resistance Exercise

INTRODUCTION

ALL GOOD EXERCISE programs for health should include a muscular fitness component. Muscular fitness generally comprises three muscular components: strength, endurance, and power. The extent to which the components of muscular fitness get developed is directly related to the exercise prescription. From a health standpoint, strength and endurance are the focus but power should not be neglected. Stressing the muscles in multiple ways can improve the force of muscle contraction, lead to longer duration of contractions before fatigue and quicker contractions. All of these improvements contribute to better balance, enhancements in activities of daily living, stronger bones, and reductions in risk for chronic diseases.

As previously mentioned, before writing exercise prescriptions, students should review the FITT-VP principles and guidelines (FITT is an acronym for Frequency, Intensity, Time, and Type of exercise; VP is an acronym for Volume and Progression).[1] For resistance training, the major focus should be on the volume of training, in particular the combination of the weights lifted, number of sets, and repetitions for each exercise. Nevertheless, the frequency, time, type, pattern, and progression must also be addressed.

The purpose of this chapter is to teach students how to design the resistance training portion of an exercise program. On completion of the case studies, students will be able to:

1. Determine the appropriate number of days per week to lift weights
2. Calculate the exercise intensity using a percent of the one-rep maximum (1-RM)
3. Recommend an appropriate number of resistance exercises that develop each of the major muscle groups
4. Establish the number of repetitions to improve strength, endurance, or power
5. Suggest the appropriate number of sets
6. Ascertain the time of rest intervals within and between workouts
7. Advise clients when to increase weights, repetitions, sets, or frequency in order to progress

COMPONENTS OF THE EXERCISE SESSION

Like cardiorespiratory training, the muscular training session should include warm-up, conditioning, cool-down, and stretching components. While the conditioning component is very different, the other components are very similar. The session should begin with less than 15 minutes of light activity. Following the conditioning component, which is described in detail below, is 5 to 10 minutes of light activity of cool-down. Ten or more minutes of stretching should be included, which generally would follow the cool-down when the muscles are still warm.

MUSCULAR FITNESS CONDITIONING

The conditioning phase for muscular fitness training uses resistance exercises. The intensity, repetitions, and sets completed determine the specific type of muscular fitness developed. Performing lower repetitions with higher intensities focuses on power. Performing moderate repetitions with moderate intensities focuses on strength. Performing higher repetitions with lower intensities focuses on endurance. For the general healthy population to maintain health the focus is usually on strength.

Frequency. Resistance training one day per week can maintain strength. However, the general recommendation is to perform resistance training exercises two or more times per week. This frequency of training will usually result in improvements.

Intensity. The recommended amount of weight to lift for the various exercises is indicated by a percent of the one-repetition maximum (1-RM). However, in practice it may not be reasonable to determine the 1-RM for each exercise. The 1-RM may be tested for a couple of major lifts such as bench press and leg press. From there it is trial and error. The actual starting weights are estimates with a focus on the prescribed number of repetitions. If at the beginning of the training the client is unable to lift the target number of repetitions the weight is reduced. If the client can do more repetitions than prescribed the weight is increased. This is done until a good resistance weight is determined for each exercise.

Generally speaking, to improve strength beginners should start with lighter weights (40%–50% of 1-RM), work up to higher weights (60%–70% of 1-RM) for novices, and then heavier weights (80+% of 1-RM) for experienced lifters. If muscular endurance is the goal then lighter weights (less than 50% 1-RM) should be used.

Type. There are many different resistance training exercises that can be performed. The important consideration is that all the major muscle groups be included. Multi-joint and single-joint exercises can be used but in terms of exercise order the multi-joint exercises for a muscle group should be done before the single-joint exercises that use the same muscle group. This is to avoid fatiguing one muscle in the group before it is worked again in the multi-joint exercise.

In terms of equipment type, anything that resists muscle contraction will work. The includes but is not limited to free weights, various weight machines, resistance bands, and exercises using the body for resistance. The important factor is that the muscles get stressed and overloaded.

Repetitions. The key variable in the resistance training exercise prescription is the number of times the weight is lifted without rest. This contributes to the type of muscular fitness that is developed most. For most people lower reps (3–6) improves power, medium reps (8–12 for untrained) improves strength, and higher reps (15–25) improves endurance. First the type of muscular fitness desired should be determined. Then the number of repetitions targeted is determined. Finally, the appropriate amount of weight to start with for each exercise can be decided.

Sets. Each resistance exercise should be done two to four times in a training session for most people to improve strength. To improve muscular endurance one or two sets can be prescribed. Beginners and older people can benefit from doing only one set. Individuals with goals to improve performance, not simply health, can benefit by completing more than four sets in some workouts each week.

Pattern. There is a rest period between sets when doing multiple sets. The typical time is two to three minutes. This will give the muscles time to recover somewhat before doing the next set. If time efficiency is important one-minute rests are acceptable.

Resistance training is intense and can deplete the muscle glycogen stores. Because it takes about two days to replenish glycogen, a 48-hour rest is recommended before working the same muscles groups again. Because the frequency of training is usually two to three times per week, the same muscle groups can be worked every other day with an extra day of rest or two each week. For those wanting to lift weights more often than three times per week the exercise sessions must be divided into areas such as upper body, lower body, and core. Each area can be worked twice per week while the other areas recover.

Progression. In order to continue improving muscular fitness at least one of the variables must be increased periodically. To increase the overload on the muscles over time the amount of resistance, number of reps, number of sets, or frequency of training must be increased. One or more of these increases should be made when the exerciser can do more reps than targeted consistently over several workouts.

Demonstration Case Study 7.1

Resistance exercise

Mac is a 20-year-old man who has been lifting weights for several years. He currently weighs 220 pounds but wants to get bigger muscles. He has been doing the same general program for two years, focusing on squats and bench press. He has tried to lift on most days. He visits a gym and talks with the exercise physiologist, Mike, about designing a better program. They do some basic paperwork and Mike determines that Mac can safely perform high-intensity exercise.

Mike begins with the FITT-VP principle for resistance exercise. He tells Mac that muscles need 48 hours to recover and he should not be lifting with the same muscle groups two days in a row. Three days per week of lifting would be a good frequency. Once Mac's body adapts to the new program they can consider adding more days per week by limiting each lifting session to certain muscle groups.

Next Mike considers the specific type of exercises to include. He wants to incorporate single-joint and multi-joint exercises that involve the major muscle groups. A combination of free weights and resistance machines is considered. Mike recommends the following exercises:

Leg press (hip and knee extensors)

Knee extension (knee extensors)

Leg curls (knee flexors)

Hip adduction (hip adductors)

Hip abduction (hip abductors)

Toe raises (ankle plantar flexors)

Bench press (elbow extensors and shoulder horizontal adductors)

Lat pull downs (elbow flexors and shoulder adductors)

Overhead press (elbow extensors and shoulder flexors)

Upright row (elbow flexors and shoulder horizontal abductors)

Biceps curls (elbow flexors)

Triceps curls (elbow extensors)

Abdominal curls (trunk flexors)

Trunk extension (trunk extensors)

Trunk rotations (trunk rotators)

Mike notes that time of training is not formally identified for resistance exercise, so he moves on the intensity, sets, and reps, which together determine the volume of training. He talks with Mac about the amount of weight he can lift and the number of reps he can do. Mike then estimates the one-rep maximum (1-RM) for each exercise. Because Mac's primary goal is to get bigger by adding more muscle mass to his body, and because he is an experienced weight lifter, Mike recommends he start at 75% of his estimated 1-RM for each exercise. Mike takes a list of the exercises and multiplies the 1-RM by 0.75 to get his recommended starting weight.

Exercise	1-RM (pounds)	Starting Weight (pounds)
Leg press	600	450
Knee extension	300	225
Leg curls	240	180
Hip adduction	300	225
Hip abduction	260	195
Toe raises	200	150
Bench press	280	210
Lat pull downs	280	210

Exercise	1-RM (pounds)	Starting Weight (pounds)
Overhead press	200	150
Upright row	200	150
Biceps curls	100	75
Triceps curls	200	150
Abdominal curls	220	165
Trunk extension	280	210
Trunk rotations	180	135

With the intensity determined Mike considers the number of reps and sets. Because Mac's goal is hypertrophy, Mike advises four sets of eight reps at the 75% of 1-RM to volitional failure.

For the lifting pattern Mike recommends no more than three-minute rest intervals between sets. He further explains that when Mac can do 10 reps of an exercise for two consecutive workouts he should increase the weight for that exercise by 5% for upper body exercises and 10% for lower body exercises in order to progress and continue to gain muscle mass and strength.

Mike then goes over the typical workout session. He advises Mac to begin his workout session with five to ten minutes on one of the cardio machines to increase the temperature of his muscles to prepare them for lifting. After getting the muscles warm he recommends about five minutes of dynamic stretching by using similar movements of the lifts planned for the workout.

Once Mac has completed the lifting workout outlined by Mike he should complete a 10-minute cool-down. Mike recommends using cardio equipment such as walking on a treadmill. This will help to maintain blood flow and clear some of the lactic acid that has accumulated in the muscles. This cool-down should be followed by 10 minutes more of static flexibility exercises.

Mac is excited about his exercise prescription and is ready to start lifting weights.

Student Case Study 7.1

Resistance exercise

Martina is a 24-year-old marathon runner who weighs 105 pounds. She has completed three marathons but has failed to make any major improvements in her times despite increasing her weekly mileage. She talks to a trainer who suggests resistance training to increase her muscular strength and endurance. Martina completes a screening and, not surprisingly, is found to be healthy and able to do strenuous exercise.

Because Martina has not lifted weights before, she completes a battery of muscular strength lifts using resistance machines rather than free weights. She is found to have the following estimated 1-RMs: leg press = 150 pounds, bench press = 60 pounds, and seated row = 60 pounds. On the push-up test she is able to complete 8 push-ups. Using the FITT-VP principle for resistance training develop Martina's exercise prescription.

1. Indicate which exercises should be performed.
2. Determine the initial intensity for each exercise.
3. Recommend the frequency of training and why.
4. Prescribe the combination of sets and reps and why they were selected.
5. Designate the rest pattern during and between exercise sessions.
6. Propose the nonconditioning components of the exercise training session.

Student Case Study 7.2

Resistance exercise

D'Angelo is a 43-year-old man who weighs 167 pounds. He has been walking 40 minutes per day for the last six years. During this time he lost 57 pounds. While his walking has been going well he has noticed that his general strength has been decreasing and he would like to begin a resistance training program. D'Angelo visits the local health and fitness club and completes a screening where he is found to be healthy and able to do strenuous exercise.

At the fitness club D'Angelo completes a fitness assessment. He is found to have the following 1-RMs: leg press = 275 pounds, bench press = 150 pounds. On the push-up test he completed 12 push-ups. Using the FITT-VP principle for resistance training, develop D'Angelo's exercise prescription.

1. Indicate which exercises should be performed.
2. Determine the initial intensity for each exercise.
3. Recommend the frequency of training and provide the reason for this.
4. Prescribe the combination of sets and reps and provide the reason they were selected.
5. Designate the rest pattern during and between exercise sessions.
6. Propose the nonconditioning components of the exercise training session.

Student Case Study 7.3

Resistance exercise

Jordann is a 30-year-old mother of two who weighs 126 pounds. After noticing that her muscles have become soft, she is looking to get back into muscular shape. She talks to a trainer who suggests resistance training to increase her muscle tone. Jordann completes a screening after which it is determined that she is healthy and safely able to do strenuous exercise.

Jordann goes to the fitness club and completes a battery of muscular tests. Her estimated 1-RMs are: leg press = 120 pounds, bench press = 65 pounds. She is able to complete 13 push-ups on the push-up test. Using the FITT-VP principle for resistance training develop Jordann's exercise prescription.

1. Indicate which exercises should be performed.
2. Determine the initial intensity for each exercise.
3. Recommend the frequency of training and provide the reason for this.
4. Prescribe the combination of sets and reps and provide the reason they were selected.
5. Designate the rest pattern during and between exercise sessions.
6. Propose the nonconditioning components of the exercise training session.

REFERENCE

1. American College of Sports Medicine. *ACSM's Guidelines for Exercise Testing and Prescription*, 11th edition. Philadelphia, PA: Wolters Kluwer Health, 2022.

CHAPTER 8

FITT-VP Principle for Flexibility Exercise

INTRODUCTION

T HOUGH FLEXIBILITY EXERCISES are not usually a major component of a general exercise program, they should be a part of all exercise programs. Flexibility is one component of fitness that can be trained daily without recovery days. When designing flexibility programs, there are several types of stretching to consider: static, dynamic, and ballistic. Each type has appropriate applications. Static stretching includes several subtypes: active, passive, and proprioceptive neuromuscular facilitation. Any type of stretching, if performed properly, can improve joint range of motion immediately and over the long term. Also, stretching can help improve posture and balance.

Like for the other components of fitness discussed previously, students should review the FITT-VP principles and guidelines before attempting the case studies. (FITT is an acronym for Frequency, Intensity, Time, and Type of exercise; VP is an acronym for Volume and Progression.) Similar to resistance training, flexibility training should focus on the total volume of training. For flexibility this includes the total time stretches are held per session multiplied by the number of sessions per week.

The purpose of this chapter is to teach students how to design the flexibility training portion of an exercise program. On completion of the case studies, students will be able to:

1. Recommend the appropriate number of days per week to stretch
2. Determine the exercise intensity or degree of the stretch
3. Decide an appropriate number of flexibility exercises that develop each of the major joints
4. Establish the total time of stretch
5. Suggest the pattern of exercises including the number of reps and ideal time during the overall workout

TYPES OF STRETCHING

If properly done, all types of flexibility exercises are effective. However, it is important to select the correct type for different people in order to maximize flexibility development and safety.

Ballistic. Increasing the stretch by using momentum developed by the fast contraction of the antagonistic muscles activates the stretch reflex. This movement provides for a good stretch of the muscle–tendon complex but too much momentum can cause too much stretch. Overstretching can cause injury and soreness. The best time to use ballistic stretching is before sport activities where ballistic movements are common. This will help to prepare for the sport movements. They must be performed properly with muscles that are warm. Ballistic stretches are not generally used by the general population exercising to improve health.

Dynamic. Slower movement stretches that engage the stretch reflex in a more controlled way can improve flexibility with less risk of overstretching. Repeating the same motion slowly and gradually increasing the range of motion with each repetition is effective. This is often done when the muscles are tight from being the same position for a while to get some flexibility back. Dynamic stretches can also be done as part of the planned stretching program. It is generally safer than ballistic stretching but not as effective as static stretching.

Static. Slowly stretching the muscle tendon complex to the point of tension and then holding that stretched position for 10 to 30 seconds is a safe and effective way to increase flexibility and range of motion. Static stretching can be done actively or passively. Active static stretching uses the contraction of the antagonist muscle to perform the stretch. Passive stretching uses assistance to perform the stretch such as from a partner or gravity. Static stretching is most commonly recommended for the general population.

Proprioceptive neuromuscular facilitation (PNF). PNF stretching is a superior set of stretches that is noted for its capability of achieving a greater range of motion in comparison to active or passive static, dynamic, or ballistic stretching techniques. PNF stretching advantageously uses certain protective proprioceptive mechanisms of the body to increase the achieved range of motion for a given stretch. Overall, PNF stretching is based on two key principles: autogenic inhibition and reciprocal inhibition.

Autogenic inhibition occurs from direct involvement of the Golgi tendon organs (GTOs), which are primarily embedded within the tendons of skeletal muscles. GTOs are a special class of proprioceptors commonly referred to as mechanoreceptors. GTOs are responsible for detecting the force generated from muscular contraction. Once stimulated, GTOs send a signal to the spinal cord resulting in the inhibition of further contraction. This particular mechanism helps guard the muscle from injury by preventing excessive muscular force generation. In PNF stretching, the muscle being targeted for the stretch is contracted, either isometrically or dynamically, for at least 6 seconds. During these 6 seconds of contraction, the GTOs are stimulated and the muscle being stretched is inhibited, to a certain extent, from further contraction. As a result, the muscle being targeted for the stretch is more relaxed and can be pushed further into the stretch, which permits greater range of motion of the stretch.

To understand reciprocal inhibition it is beneficial to have some basic knowledge of neuromuscular anatomy. Motor neurons originate in the spinal cord and are responsible for innervating skeletal muscles. In the spinal cord motor neurons split. One branch travels to an agonist muscle and another to the antagonist muscle. When a motor neuron sends an excitatory signal (a signal for muscular contraction) to an agonist muscle, its split division will send an inhibitory signal to the antagonist muscle. Thus, when an agonist muscle contracts and shortens, the antagonist muscle relaxes to permit a joint movement. Therefore, a common PNF stretching technique calls for the contraction of the antagonist muscle group to elicit relaxation in the muscle being stretched. An example of this is contracting the quadriceps muscle for hip flexion to stretch the hamstring muscles. Whenever this type of PNF stretching technique is used, the stretch is relying on reciprocal inhibition to achieve a greater range of motion during the stretch.

PNF stretching most frequently involves a partner stretch protocol. These protocols are hold–relax, contract–relax, and hold–relax with antagonist contraction. The first two of these protocols rely on autogenic inhibition while the third relies on both autogenic and reciprocal inhibition. These protocols are described next.

Hold–Relax

a. First a partner will passively "pre-stretch" the joint. Here the partner moves the joint as far into the stretch as possible (without pain) and holds for 10 seconds.

b. After 10 seconds, the partner instructs the person being stretched to resist the attempt to move the stretch further. This is done for 6 seconds.

c. After resistance, the partner will instruct the person being stretched to relax and then the partner will move the stretch forward as far as possible and hold for 30 seconds.

Contract–Relax

a. First a partner will passively "pre-stretch" the joint. Here the partner moves the joint as far into the stretch as possible (without pain) and holds for 10 seconds.

b. After 10 seconds, the partner instructs the person being stretched to concentrically contract against resistance. The partner will allow full contraction, throughout a range of motion, slowly.

c. After contraction, the partner will move the joint into the range of motion as far as possible and hold for 30 seconds.

Hold–Relax with Antagonist Contraction

a. First a partner will passively "pre-stretch" the joint. Here the partner moves the joint as far into the stretch as possible (without pain) and holds for 10 seconds.

b. After 10 seconds, the partner instructs the person being stretched to resist their attempt to move the stretch further. This is done for 6 seconds.

c. After resistance, the partner instructs the person being stretched to assist the stretch by actively moving into the range of motion. The stretch is held for 30 seconds.

IMPROVING FLEXIBILITY

Stretching exercises should be a part of all exercise sessions. Stretching after the warm-up or cool-down will help to improve overall flexibility. However, if greater improvements are desired a stand-alone flexibility session can be done. To make improvements in flexibility the FITT-VP principles should be followed.[1]

Frequency. Stretching exercises should be done at least two times per week. The more frequently stretching is performed the better. Stretching can be done daily, though other types of training should not be performed daily. Because stretching is recommended as part of every exercise session it should be done every workout day.

Intensity. It is important to get a good stretch without stretching too far. To gauge intensity the stretch should be to the point of mild discomfort, but never pain.

Time. How long a stretch should be held depends on the type of stretch done. Ballistic and dynamic stretches are not held. Static stretches are held for 10 to 30 seconds. Older exercisers may hold static stretches to 1 minute. PNF stretches are held for various times depending on the type done.

Type. All types of stretching are effective if done properly. Static and PNF are most widely used for the general population. When writing the exercise prescription it is important to include all the major muscle tendon complexes.

Volume. The general recommendation is to hold each stretch for a total of 90 seconds. For example, a stretch can be done three times and held for 30 seconds or done two times and held for 45 seconds. Other combinations are acceptable. Because stretches are not held in ballistic and dynamic exercises this guideline cannot be effectively used.

Pattern. It is always recommended that stretching exercises be performed while the body is warm. Cold stretching can more likely result in injuries and shorter stretching through the range of motion. Each exercise should be done two to four times but that depends on the time for which the stretch is held.

Demonstration Case Study 8.1

Flexibility exercise

Kiana is a 19-year-old college sophomore. She has been lifting weights and using cardio machines in the university recreation center for the last year. She has markedly improved her cardiorespiratory endurance and muscular strength. However, she has noticed that her muscles have become very tight. One day at the rec center she meets with an exercise physiologist, Marco. He assesses Kiana's flexibility with a goniometer and finds her flexibility is below average. He then outlines a stretching program for her using the FITT-VP for flexibility exercise.

Marco begins with frequency and recommends that Kiana stretch after the cool-down for each cardiorespiratory training or resistance training workout. On days she does not train he recommends that she still does the stretching program after a brief warm-up. Marco recommends the following static stretches:

Straight arms behind back (anterior deltoid, pectoralis major)

Side bend with bent arms (external oblique, latissimus dorsi, serratus anterior, triceps)

Cross arms in front of chest (posterior deltoid, rhomboids, middle trapezius)

Spinal twist (internal and external obliques, piriformis, erector spinae)

Siting toe touch (hamstrings, erector spinae, gastrocnemius)

Butterfly (hip adductors, sartorius)

Side quadriceps stretch (quadriceps, iliopsoas)

Wall stretch (gastrocnemius, soleus)

Marco further says that after she improves her flexibility he will vary the static stretches and incorporate some dynamic stretches.

For intensity and time Marco instructs Kiana to do each stretch to the point of slight discomfort and hold the stretch for 30 seconds. For volume he advises 90 seconds total time for each stretch, therefore repeating each stretch three times.

Student Case Study 8.1

Flexibility exercise

Mark is a 56-year-old man who has been doing static-stretching exercises as part of his overall exercise program. He does a few exercises he learned from a friend. He does each exercise three or four times and holds the stretch for about 10 seconds. His muscles feel very tight and he does not think the exercises he does are doing the job. Using the FITT-VP for flexibility exercise, redesign Mark's stretching program.

1. Identify the flexibility exercises to include in the prescription.
2. Indicate the type of stretch to be used: static, dynamic, etc.
3. State how often stretching should be done.
4. Define the intensity of stretching to be used.
5. Designate the time for each stretch.
6. Determine the volume of stretching to be done.
7. Outline the pattern of the stretching routine.

Student Case Study 8.2

Flexibility exercise

Lauren is a 17-year-old woman who plays recreational soccer and basketball. Her soccer coach has the team do static stretching before practice and games. She heard from a friend who plays on the high school varsity soccer team that static stretching temporarily reduces power, which can negatively affect performance in soccer. Using the FITT-VP, design a dynamic stretching program for Lauren.

1. Identify the flexibility exercises to include in the prescription.
2. Indicate the type of stretch to be used: static, dynamic, etc.
3. State how often stretching should be done.
4. Define the intensity of stretching to be used.
5. Designate the time for each stretch.
6. Determine the volume of stretching to be done.
7. Outline the pattern of the stretching routine.

REFERENCE

1. American College of Sports Medicine. *ACSM's Guidelines for Exercise Testing and Prescription*, 11th edition. Philadelphia, PA: Wolters Kluwer Health, 2022.

CHAPTER 9

FITT-VP Principle for Special Considerations

INTRODUCTION

SOME GROUPS WITHIN the healthy population require special considerations when applying the FITT-VP principles for cardiorespiratory, resistance, and flexibility training. These groups include children and adolescents, older adults, and women who are pregnant.

Children and adolescents include those who have not reached puberty. One major concern is the underdeveloped skeleton cannot tolerate as high loads as the adult skeleton. Also, because of their lower anaerobic capacities children cannot perform vigorous activities for as long a time as adults.

Older adults generally include individuals who are 65 years and older or those 50 to 64 years old who have limitations for movement and physical activity. Although older adults obtain many of the same benefits from exercise as younger adults, modifications in the exercise prescription must be considered. The intensity of exercise may need to be reduced in some cases and this reduction may be offset by increased frequency of exercise or increased workout time.

Healthy, fit women who are pregnant can tolerate exercise well. However, there are a few modifications to a workout program that should be considered, with a focus on an appropriate exercise volume depending on pre-pregnancy exercise habits. In general, exercise intensity is often decreased for women who have not previously exercised to maintain recommended frequency and duration.

Before students attempt the case studies they must review and understand the FITT-VP principles and guidelines for each component of fitness and identified population.[1] (FITT is an acronym for Frequency, Intensity, Time, and Type of exercise; VP is an acronym for Volume and Progression.) Although the FITT-VP guidelines are similar to those for the general population there are clear special considerations for writing the exercise prescriptions. It is recommended that since students have already learned the general FITT-VP principles they learn the slight variations that are appropriate for each group.

The purpose of this chapter is to teach students how to design the overall exercise program taking into consideration these special considerations. On completion of the case studies, students will be able to:

1. Adapt the general FITT-VP principles to the following groups:
    a. Children and adolescents
    b. Older adults
    c. Pregnant women
2. Write the exercise prescription considering the following components of fitness:
    a. Cardiorespiratory exercise
    b. Resistance training
    c. Flexibility exercise
3. Identify modifications needed for the exercise session

CHILDREN AND ADOLESCENTS

Clearly the youngest people should participate in planned physical activity, like those in other age groups. However, children and adolescents have very different needs and risks. As people age, the risk of cardiac events increases. For the younger age groups this is less of a concern, although congenital heart problems can be an issue. The bigger concern for those who have yet to reach maturity is bone development and growth. The growth plates in the long bones have yet to fuse, making them more susceptible to injury. Therefore activities that place high stresses on the bone should be avoided. However, bone growth responds to stresses on the bone and moderate stress should be encouraged.

Prescribing exercise for children and adolescents is not as specific as for adults. They should participate in physical activities for at least one hour every day. These activities should include aerobic, resistance, and bone strengthening exercises. Cardiovascular fitness activities should be fun and include running, fast walking, swimming, bicycling, and sports that increase heart rate and breathing at least three times per week.

Resistance exercises should also be done at least three times per week and include unstructured play, which uses the body's weight for resistance or structured resistance training using weights or bands. The focus on resistance training should be proper form and lower resistances (intensity) to avoid bone and joint injuries.

Some of the aforementioned activities can also contribute to bone strengthening and should be done three days per week. Bone strengthening activities include those that involve running, jumping, and resistance training.

In addition to the recommended physical activities mentioned earlier, children and adolescents should avoid extended sedentary time, particularly screen time. Even those who participate in the minimum one hour per day of physical activity following the guidelines listed above and spend hours per day in sedentary activities will have increased health risks and inadequate development of good lifestyle health habits.

OLDER ADULTS

Physical fitness in general declines with age and those who are older have much to gain from exercise programs. While most of the guidelines for the typical healthy population apply to older adults there are some intentional differences. For aerobic exercise the intensity prescriptions are often made using the 10-point perceived exertion scale rather than heart rates. Moderate intensity is 5 to 6 on the scale and vigorous intensity is 7 to 8. Frequency and time are 30 to 60 minutes per day, at least five times per week for moderate intensity activities and 20 to 30 minutes per day, three to five times per week for vigorous intensity activities. The type of activity is continuous and rhythmical, which does not complicate any musculoskeletal or other health problems.

Resistance training is recommended at least two times per week to help maintain bone density and muscle mass. Lower weights (beginning at 40%–50% 1-RM) are recommended with higher repetitions (beginning with 10–15 reps). Progression to 60% to 80% of the one-rep maximum is encouraged as older adults adapt to resistance training. Power training is also recommended using lower weights (30%–60% 1-RM) and completing one to three sets of six to ten repetitions at high, controlled velocities. Flexibility recommendations mirror those for the general population with a focus on static stretching.

Because people tend to have more balance problems as they age, some older adults may benefit from neuromotor training. In terms of the FITT-VP principles there is not much consensus on the standards. Generally two to three workouts per week of 20 to 30 minutes is beneficial. Tai chi and yoga are good types of classes to improve neuromotor skills.

PREGNANT WOMEN

Women who have been exercising in the past can continue to exercise after becoming pregnant as long as no complications develop. Although it would be wise to start an exercise program before becoming pregnant sedentary women can begin to exercise after pregnancy. In either case, women should be screened for physical activity and a physician approval should be obtained. The PARmed-X for Pregnancy[2] should be completed. Sections A and B, which include past pregnancy and exercise information, should be completed by the pregnant woman and Section C, which includes the contraindications to exercise, by her physician. The physician will determine if physical activity is recommended.

There are several governments or organizations that provide exercise prescription recommendations for pregnant women. They all agree to using perceived exertion instead of heart rate to monitor aerobic exercise intensity and to include muscle strengthening exercises. General guidelines include accumulating 150 minutes per week of moderate-intensity exercise.

Special considerations for pregnant women must be considered when participating in exercise programs. Exercises done while lying on the back should be avoided after the 16th week of pregnancy. In this position and at this time of pregnancy the fetus places sufficient weight on the ascending vena cava to restrict the venous return and cardiac output. The Valsalva maneuver should especially be avoided during pregnancy and the muscle pump should be maintained to avoid blood pooling and hypotension.

Demonstration Case Study 9.1

Special considerations: Children and adolescents

Jeromy is a 9-year-old boy who comes from a family with a history of obesity. His parents are concerned about his long-term health and want to make sure he gets regular physical activity. Unfortunately, he does not like organized team sports and would prefer to play video games. Because his parents train with a certified exercise physiologist at the YMCA, they arranged for their trainer, Susan to meet with all three of them to develop a plan.

Susan first explains that Jeromy's growing body does not need a rigid exercise prescription. What he does need is 60 minutes of physical activity every day that should include a combination of aerobic, resistance, and bone strengthening exercises. Aerobic exercise should be done daily at a moderate level that increases heart rate and breathing, such as fast walking. On at least three of those days he should do vigorous exercise with considerable increases in heart rate and breathing, such as running or fast bicycling. His muscles should be worked out with structured or unstructured activities that cause his muscles to contract multiple times and ways at least three times per week. Finally, he needs to include some activities that put stress on his bones to make them stronger. This should include running and jumping activities at least three times per week.

With Susan's guidance the family decides that every day after dinner they will go on a 30-minute family walk. Jeromy decides that he will begin skipping rope three times per week for 20 minutes. This will develop his bone strength as well as increase his heart rate and breathing. Also, Jeromy says he will join the Kids Fitness Club, which meets three times per week for one hour. This program combines running and climbing games with resistance training using elastic bands. This plan will meet the minimum 60 minutes per day of physical activity. Jeromy agrees he will also ride his bike regularly to help make up time from any missed activities.

Demonstration Case Study 9.2

Special considerations: Older adults

Ervin is a 66-year-old healthy man who just retired from a long career in real estate. Although he got some physical activity on the job when he was looking over properties he never participated in a planned exercise program. After his annual physical with

Dr. Jones, he was given a clean bill of health and was advised to begin a moderate exercise program to productively use his retirement time. Because he will have much more free time in retirement, Ervin agrees and joins a health and fitness club in his community. On his first visit he meets with Steve, an exercise physiologist.

Steve recommends a comprehensive exercise program that includes aerobic, resistance, and flexibility exercises. Because Ervin is older, Steve also recommends he do some neuromotor training. He develops the exercise prescription using the FITT-VP principle.

For aerobic fitness Steve suggests walking or cardio equipment that will be easier on his joints. Moderate-intensity exercise should be done at least five days per week. Because Ervin is older than 65 years, Steve uses the 0–10 physical exertion scale rather than a heart rate prescription. He explains to Ervin that he should work at an intensity that he rates as 5–6 on the scale. Steve further explains that in the beginning Ervin should exercise for 30 minutes continuously. If he cannot go that long continuously then he can break the 30 minutes into intervals of at least 10 minutes, but preferably longer. Once Ervin gets comfortable with the aerobic part of the program he can increase either the frequency or the time of exercise.

Next Steve addresses resistance training. He suggests Ervin lift weights twice per week to start. Because he belongs to the health and fitness club he will use the equipment available there. Steve wants to start Ervin on light resistances of about 50% of his estimated 1-RM. He starts Ervin with minimal weight to see how many reps he can do. The target is 10 reps done in sets of three. Through trial and error, Steve varies the weights with each set until Ervin can accomplish 10 reps at a moderate intensity 5–6 on the 10-point intensity scale. The following exercises are recommended:

> Leg press (hip and knee extensors)
>
> Knee extension (knee extensors)
>
> Leg curls (knee flexors)
>
> Toe raises (ankle plantar flexors)
>
> Bench press (elbow extensors and shoulder horizontal adductors)
>
> Lat pull downs (elbow flexors and shoulder adductors)
>
> Overhead press (elbow extensors and shoulder flexors)
>
> Upright row (elbow flexors and shoulder horizontal abductors)
>
> Biceps curls (elbow flexors)
>
> Triceps curls (elbow extensors)

In addition Steve proposes Ervin do some core exercises that include curl-ups and planks. To start he should do as many curl-ups as comfortable (5–6 on the 10-point scale) and planks as long as he can hold the proper position. The number and time will be increased as his body adapts.

The third major component of the exercise prescription is flexibility training. To minimize the stress on the muscle–tendon complex, Steve advises Ervin to do static stretching for 10 minutes after each resistance-training workout by doing the following stretches:

Neck rotations (sternocleidomastoid)

Neck flexion and extension (sternocleidomastoid, suboccipitals, splenae)

Straight arms behind back (anterior deltoid, pectoralis major)

Cross arm in front of chest (posterior deltoid, rhomboids, middle trapezius)

Straight arms above the head (latissimus dorsi)

Side bend with straight arms (external oblique, latissimus dorsi, serratus anterior)

Spinal twist (internal and external obliques, piriformis, erector spinae)

Siting toe touch (hamstrings, erector spinae, gastrocnemius)

Butterfly (hip adductors, sartorius)

Side quadriceps stretch (quadriceps, iliopsoas)

Step stretch (gastrocnemius, soleus)

Steve instructs Ervin to stretch to the point of slight discomfort and hold the stretch for 30 seconds. Each stretch should be done this way three times for a total stretch time of 90 seconds.

Because Ervin is getting on in years, Steve also recommends he do some neuromotor exercises to help with his balance and minimize falls as he ages. The health and fitness club offers yoga and tai chi classes as part of the membership fee. Because Ervin is retired and has some extra time, Steve says doing either one two to three times per week would be a beneficial addition to his overall workout program.

Demonstration Case Study 9.3

Special considerations: Pregnant women

Tammy is a healthy, 31-year-old woman who has been physically active for years. She just learned she is pregnant for the first time and wants to do all she can to deliver a healthy baby. She knows exercise is good for her and the fetus but wants to know more about what is appropriate in terms of exercising while pregnant. She belongs to a health and fitness club and decides to talk with one of the staff there.

McKenzie is an exercise physiologist at the health and fitness club and she meets with Tammy. She first gives Tammy a copy of the *PARmed-X for Pregnancy* and has her complete Sections A and B. Tammy answers "no" to all the "yes/no" questions and outlines her current exercise habits. McKenzie looks it over for completeness and tells Tammy she needs to have her health care provider complete Section C and sign the form. She should return the completed form to McKenzie to keep on file.

As Tammy has been exercising regularly, McKenzie plans to modify her existing program. Tammy has been walking at a moderate intensity for five times per week.

Her current heart rate prescription is 118–142 beats per minute. McKenzie explains that the heart rate prescription does not always work well during pregnancy and Tammy should monitor her work intensity using the 6–20 perceived exertion scale. McKenzie recommends using a perceived exertion of 13–14 for her walking workout. She should walk continuously for 30 minutes, five times per week.

Tammy has also been lifting weights to exhaustion three times per week. McKenzie explains it would be good to make a few changes. Three times per week would still be tolerable but she should now lift only to the point of moderate fatigue. She is presently doing two sets of eight reps. Because the intensity is being decreased, McKenzie recommends to try increasing the sets to three and reps to 10. The following exercises are recommended:

Leg press (hip and knee extensors)

Knee extension (knee extensors)

Leg curls (knee flexors)

Hip adduction (hip adductors)

Hip abduction (hip abductors)

Toe raises (ankle plantar flexors)

Bench press (elbow extensors and shoulder horizontal adductors)

Lat pull downs (elbow flexors and shoulder adductors)

Overhead press (elbow extensors and shoulder flexors)

Upright row (elbow flexors and shoulder horizontal abductors)

Biceps curls (elbow flexors)

Triceps curls (elbow extensors)

Abdominal curls (trunk flexors)

Trunk extension (trunk extensors)

Trunk rotations (trunk rotators)

McKenzie notes that it is important to use the upright bench press and upright abdominal curl machines because soon (at 16 weeks of pregnancy) she will want to avoid doing any exercises in the supine position. When lying on the back the weight of the fetus can restrict her venous return and decrease her cardiac output.

The program should also include flexibility exercises. Tammy has been doing a combination of static and dynamic flexibility exercises two to three times per week. McKenzie recommends limiting the exercises to static during the pregnancy in order to maintain better control of the movements. The following exercises are recommended:

Neck rotations (sternocleidomastoid)

Neck flexion and extension (sternocleidomastoid, suboccipitals, splenae)

Straight arms behind back (anterior deltoid, pectoralis major)

Side bend with bent arms (external oblique, latissimus dorsi, serratus anterior, triceps)

Cross arms in front of chest (posterior deltoid, rhomboids, middle trapezius)

Spinal twist (internal and external obliques, piriformis, erector spinae)

Siting toe touch (hamstrings, erector spinae, gastrocnemius)

Butterfly (hip adductors, sartorius)

Side quadriceps stretch (quadriceps, iliopsoas)

Wall stretch (gastrocnemius, soleus)

As with the resistance exercises McKenzie warns about doing stretches while lying on the back, such as the supine knee flex. The proposed stretches should be done at least three times per week after her resistance exercises. However, it would be better to do her stretching on more days such as after her cardiorespiratory workouts as well.

Tammy agrees this is a workable program. Her plan is to lift weights on Mondays, Wednesdays, and Fridays. She will do her cardio workouts on the same three days as well as on Tuesdays and Saturdays. Tammy will stretch at the end of her workouts on each cardiorespiratory and resistance workout day.

Student Case Study 9.1

Special considerations: Children and adolescents

Mia is an 8-year-old girl who is very physically active. She loves to play soccer and will play almost any physical-type games with the neighborhood kids. She plays on an organized soccer team. Her physically active parents are very happy with her interest in being active. They want to support her but not push her so hard that she burns out.

Her parents take Mia to a fitness facility to meet with an exercise physiologist. They explain that Mia would like to be a serious soccer player in the near future but they are also interested in her developing a life-long interest in exercise for health. Using the FITT principles for cardiorespiratory, resistance, and flexibility training, design an exercise program to meet Mia's goals.

1. Indicate the types of aerobic exercise to be performed.
2. Determine the intensity of aerobic exercise.
3. Recommend the time and frequency of aerobic exercise.
4. Specify the resistance exercises to be completed.
5. Establish intensity of the resistance exercises.
6. Prescribe the time and frequency of the resistance training program.
7. Identify the bone strengthening exercises to include.
8. Suggest the time and frequency of bone strengthening activities.

Student Case Study 9.2

Special considerations: Older adults

Emma is a 67-year-old woman. One year ago she fell and broke her hip. After her hospital recovery and physical therapy she is now 100% healthy. She wants to avoid future falls as much as possible and learned from her physical therapist that beginning a regular exercise program is her best insurance against falling. In her most recent physical exam her physician cleared her for participation in moderate exercise. Emma has never participated in regular physical activity in the past. Prescribe an exercise program to meet Emma's needs using the FITT principles.

1. Indicate the types of aerobic exercise to be performed.
2. Determine the intensity of aerobic exercise.
3. Recommend the time and frequency of aerobic exercise.
4. Specify the resistance exercises to be completed.
5. Establish intensity of the resistance exercises.
6. Prescribe the time and frequency of the resistance training program.
7. Identify the flexibility exercises to include.
8. Determine the intensity of stretching.
9. Suggest the time and frequency of flexibility activities.
10. Indicate any other exercise types that could be beneficial.

Student Case Study 9.3

Special considerations: Pregnant women

Lori is a 29-year-old pregnant woman. She has been running marathons since she was 20 years old. Owing to her intense training, Lori is very fit and annually improves her marathon times. She has spent the last year and a half trying to become pregnant and just found out she is expecting. She goes to her first appointment with her physician and she completes the *PARmed-X for Pregnancy*. Her physician approves Lori for physical activity.

Knowing that she will have to modify her exercise program during her pregnancy Lori decides to consult the exercise physiologist at the fitness club where she trains. Lori wants to stay in good shape during the pregnancy because she would like to start marathon training again soon after delivery. Develop her training program using the FITT principles for cardiorespiratory, resistance, and flexibility training.

1. Indicate the types of aerobic exercise to be performed.
2. Determine the intensity of aerobic exercise.
3. Recommend the time and frequency of aerobic exercise.
4. Specify the resistance exercises to be completed.

5. Establish intensity of the resistance exercises.
6. Prescribe the time and frequency of the resistance training program.
7. Identify the flexibility exercises to include.
8. Determine the intensity of stretching.
9. Suggest the time and frequency of flexibility activities.

REFERENCE

1. American College of Sports Medicine. *ACSM's Guidelines for Exercise Testing and Prescription*, 11th edition. Philadelphia, PA: Wolters Kluwer Health, 2022.

2. Canadian Society for Exercise Physiology. PARmed-X for Pregnancy, http://www.csep.ca/cmfiles/publications/parq/parmed-xpreg.pdf, 2015.

CHAPTER 10

Comprehensive Case Studies

INTRODUCTION

T HE PREVIOUS CHAPTERS have covered the steps to follow in order to write effective exercise prescriptions. Each chapter focused on one component of the process. In this last chapter students will have the opportunity to consolidate all of the concepts learned into an all-inclusive case study. This will prepare students to work with clients in the future by practicing how to design an individual exercise program from the initial screening through the final exercise prescription.

The purpose of this chapter is to teach students how to design the overall exercise program using the FITT-VP (FITT is an acronym for Frequency, Intensity, Time, and Type of exercise; VP is an acronym for Volume and Progression.) principles for cardio-respiratory endurance, resistance, and flexibility training as well as the design of the exercise session. On completion of the case studies, students will be able to:

1. Screen participants for safe exercise
2. Evaluate the risk for disease
3. Utilize metabolic equations in exercise prescription when appropriate
4. Apply the FITT-VP principle to cardiovascular endurance training
5. Apply the FITT-VP principle to resistance training
6. Apply the FITT-VP principle flexibility training
7. Integrate all types of training into a single program
8. Design the workout session to include warm-up, cool-down, and conditioning
9. Address the specific needs of special populations

Student Case Study 10.1

Comprehensive exercise prescription

Ed is a 63-year-old man who is beginning to think about retirement. He gets limited physical activity because he sits at a desk most of the day and has no regular exercise program. Despite his sedentary lifestyle he is generally healthy. He has never smoked, has no known chronic diseases and has no signs or symptoms of chronic disease but is concerned about his balance, as he stumbles frequently and is afraid of falling. Knowing that he is going to have more free time in retirement, he wants to begin an exercise program now to make his transition easier. He goes to the local fitness center where you work and inquires about membership options. Per club policy all new members are required to complete the PAR-Q+. You give him the first page of the PAR-Q+ and he answers "no" to all seven questions.

One of the reasons Ed wants to start exercising is because his father had a fatal heart attack at the age of 62 years before he was able to retire. His father had previous heart attacks at 54 and 60 years of age. His mother is still living at 86 years of age. His two siblings are currently healthy. As part of his physical exam it was found that Ed is 6 feet tall and weighs 209 pounds. His resting heart rate is 70 beats per minute and his resting blood pressure is 132/80 mm Hg. His blood test showed his LDL-C = 108 mg/dL, HDL-C = 29 mg/dL, and fasting plasma glucose = 90 mg/dL.

Ed completes a fitness assessment that includes a submax modified YMCA cycle ergometer test. The test results were:

- chest skinfolds = 12 mm
- triceps skinfold = 18 mm
- thigh skinfold = 11 mm
- subscapular skinfold = 20 mm
- midaxillary skinfold = 15 mm
- abdomen subscapular skinfold = 36 mm
- suprailiac skinfold = 38 mm
- right hand grip strength = 49 kg
- left hand grip strength = 46 kg
- leg press 1-RM = 410 pounds
- bench press 1-RM = 165 pounds
- push-ups = 19
- hip flexion range of motion = 124 degrees
- countermovement vertical jump = 17 cm

Submax modified YMCA cycle ergometer test results using a Monark ergometer were:

Stage	Minute of Test	Heart Rate Beats/min	Blood Pressure mm Hg	Resistance kg	Workload kg-m/min	Other
I	1	84		0.5	150	
I	2	96		0.5	150	
I	3	96	142/80	0.5	150	
II	4	108		1.5	450	
II	5	112		1.5	450	
II	6	114	150/82	1.5	450	
III	7	122		2.0	600	
III	8	128		2.0	600	
III	9	130	158/82	2.0	600	2 heart rates > 110 bpm

1. Does he need to complete pages 2 and 3 of the PAR-Q+, and why or why not?
2. Does he need to complete the ePARmed-X+, and why or why not?
3. Based on the PAR-Q+, can he begin the exercise program? Why or why not?
4. Based on the PAR-Q+, can he perform moderate or vigorous exercise to start? Why?
5. Based on the American College of Sports Medicine (ACSM) Pre-participation Screening Algorithm, should he get medical clearance before beginning? Why or why not?
6. Based on the ACSM Pre-participation Screening Algorithm, can he perform moderate or vigorous exercise? Why or why not?
7. Based on the ACSM Pre-participation Screening Algorithm, should he get medical clearance before progressing to higher intensities? Why or why not?
8. What are the positive risk factors for cardiovascular disease (CVD)?
9. What are the negative risk factors for CVD?
10. Which risk factors does the client not have?
11. How many risk factors does the client have?
12. What lifestyle changes would you recommend? Why?
13. Determine his pre-test likelihood of ischemic heart disease.
14. Determine the exercise heart rate at which the test should be stopped if reached.
15. Calculate his percent body fat and fitness category.
16. Determine his estimated maximum oxygen consumption $(\dot{V}O_{2max})$ by extrapolating the test data and determine his percentile classification.
17. Evaluate his hand grip strength score and fitness category.
18. Determine his fitness category for the bench press and leg press.
19. Find his fitness category for the push-up test.
20. Rate his hip flexion range of motion (average, below average or above average).
21. Determine his fitness category for the vertical jump.
22. Calculate a heart rate prescription using the heart rate reserve method.
23. Calculate the prescription using the $\dot{V}O_2$ reserve method.
24. Compute the resistance he should use when riding a Monark cycle ergometer at 50 rpm using the midpoint of the $\dot{V}O_2$ reserve method.
25. Figure out how many calories he would burn on the cycle ergometer if he cycled for 30 minutes.
26. Indicate which exercise group should be used for the type of exercise as well as the frequency and time of exercise.
27. Verify if the prescription is the appropriate volume and comment on the pattern and progression.
28. Design the make-up of the entire aerobic exercise session.
29. Develop his resistance training prescription considering which exercises he should do, initial intensity, frequency, sets, reps, and pattern.
30. Design the nonconditioning components of the exercise resistance training session.
31. Using the FITT-VP for flexibility exercise design his stretching program.

32. What additional exercise would be recommended for his balance and why?

Comprehensive exercise prescription

Mary is a 26-year-old woman who is looking forward to getting married and having children. For the last four years she has worked for a management consulting firm and has worked very long hours that included much travel. She just changed jobs and now can settle into a 40-hour workweek. Her plan is to use her extra time to increase her exercise time. Although she has been using cardio machines at low intensity for an average of 30 minutes, two times per week in the hotel fitness rooms she wants to get more consistent cardio workouts and add resistance training. She never smoked, has no known chronic diseases and has no signs or symptoms of chronic disease. She goes to the health and fitness club that is available to employees at her new job. Per company policy all new members are required to complete the PAR-Q+. You give her the first page of the PAR-Q+ and he answers "no" to all seven questions.

Mary's parents are in their mid 50s and healthy. During her physical exam it was established that Mary is 5 feet 3 inches tall and weighs 248 pounds. Her resting heart rate is 69 beats per minute and her resting blood pressure is 114/72 mm Hg. Her blood test found her LDL-C = 96 mg/dL, HDL-C = 32 mg/dL, and fasting plasma glucose = 94 mg/dL.

Mary completes a fitness assessment that includes the Queens College Step Test. The test results were:

- triceps skinfold = 16 mm
- subscapular skinfold = 18 mm
- midaxillary skinfold = 14 mm
- abdomen subscapular skinfold = 29 mm
- suprailiac skinfold = 31 mm
- right hand grip strength = 27 kg
- left hand grip strength = 25 kg
- leg press 1-RM = 220 pounds
- bench press 1-RM = 110 pounds
- push-ups = 13
- hip flexion range of motion = 135 degrees
- countermovement vertical jump = 28 cm

The single-stage Queens College Step Test was performed at 22 steps per minute for 3 minutes. Her 15-second heart rate was 42 beats.

1. Does she need to complete pages 2 and 3 of the PAR-Q+, and why or why not?
2. Does she need to complete the ePARmed-X+, and why or why not?
3. Based on the PAR-Q+, can she begin the exercise program? Why or why not?

4. Based on the PAR-Q+, should she perform moderate or vigorous exercise to start? Why?
5. Based on the ACSM Pre-participation Screening Algorithm, should she get medical clearance before beginning? Why or why not?
6. Based on the ACSM Pre-participation Screening Algorithm, can she perform moderate or vigorous exercise? Why?
7. Based on the ACSM Pre-participation Screening Algorithm, should she get medical clearance before progressing to higher intensities? Why or why not?
8. What are the positive risk factors for CVD?
9. What are the negative risk factors for CVD?
10. Which risk factors does the client not have?
11. How many risk factors does the client have?
12. What lifestyle changes would you recommend? Why?
13. Determine her pre-test likelihood of ischemic heart disease.
14. Calculate her percent body fat and fitness category.
15. Estimate her $\dot{V}O_{2max}$ from the step test and determine her percentile classification.
16. Evaluate her hand grip strength score and fitness category.
17. Determine her fitness category for the bench press and leg press.
18. Find her fitness category for the push-up test.
19. Rate her hip flexion range of motion (average, below average or above average).
20. Determine her fitness category for the vertical jump.
21. Calculate a heart rate prescription using the heart rate reserve method.
22. Calculate the prescription using the $\dot{V}O_2$ reserve method.
23. Compute how fast she should walk/run on a treadmill at 5% grade using the midpoint of the $\dot{V}O_2$ reserve method.
24. Figure how many calories she would burn on the treadmill if she exercised for 40 minutes.
25. Indicate which aerobic exercise group should be used for the type of exercise as well as the frequency and time of exercise.
26. Verify if the prescription is the appropriate volume and comment on the pattern and progression.
27. Design the make-up of the entire aerobic exercise session.
28. Develop her resistance training prescription considering which exercises she should do, initial intensity, frequency, sets, reps, and pattern.
29. Design the nonconditioning components of the exercise resistance training session.
30. Using the FITT-VP for flexibility exercise design her stretching program.